50 Studies Every Internist Should Know

50 STUDIES EVERY DOCTOR SHOULD KNOW

Published and Forthcoming Books in the *50 Studies Every Doctor Should Know* Series

50 Studies Every Doctor Should Know: The Key Studies That Form the Foundation of Evidence Based Medicine, Revised Edition
Michael E. Hochman

50 Studies Every Internist Should Know
Edited by Kristopher Swiger, Joshua R. Thomas, Michael E. Hochman, and Steven D. Hochman

50 Studies Every Neurologist Should Know
Edited by David Y. Hwang and David M. Greer

50 Studies Every Surgeon Should Know
Edited by SreyRam Kuy and Rachel J. Kwon

50 Studies Every Pediatrician Should Know
Edited by Ashaunta Tumblin, Nina L. Shapiro, Stephen C. Aronoff, Jeremiah Davis, and Michael Levy

50 Imaging Studies Every Doctor Should Know
Christoph Lee

50 Studies Every Anesthesiologist Should Know
Anita Gupta

Interested in writing or proposing a book in the series?
Email: fiftystudies@gmail.com

50 Studies Every Internist Should Know

EDITED BY

Kristopher J. Swiger, MD

Resident Physician, Internal Medicine
The Johns Hopkins Hospital
Baltimore, Maryland

Joshua R. Thomas, MD, MPH

Cardiology Fellow, Pediatrics and Adult Congenital HD
Nationwide Children's Hospital
The Ohio State University
Columbus, Ohio

Michael E. Hochman, MD, MPH

Medical Director for Innovation
AltaMed Health Services
Los Angeles, California

Steven D. Hochman, MPH

Medical Student
Keck School of Medicine of the University of Southern California
Los Angeles, California

SERIES EDITOR:

Michael E. Hochman, MD, MPH

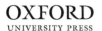

OXFORD
UNIVERSITY PRESS

OXFORD

UNIVERSITY PRESS

Oxford University Press is a department of the University of
Oxford. It furthers the University's objective of excellence in research,
scholarship, and education by publishing worldwide.

Oxford New York

Auckland Cape Town Dar es Salaam Hong Kong Karachi
Kuala Lumpur Madrid Melbourne Mexico City Nairobi
New Delhi Shanghai Taipei Toronto

With offices in

Argentina Austria Brazil Chile Czech Republic France Greece
Guatemala Hungary Italy Japan Poland Portugal Singapore
South Korea Switzerland Thailand Turkey Ukraine Vietnam

Oxford is a registered trademark of Oxford University Press
in the UK and certain other countries.

Published in the United States of America by
Oxford University Press
198 Madison Avenue, New York, NY 10016

© Oxford University Press 2015

Library of Congress Cataloging-in-Publication Data
50 studies every internist should know / edited by Kristopher J. Swiger, Joshua R. Thomas,
Michael E. Hochman, Steven D. Hochman.
    p. ; cm. — (50 studies every doctor should know)
50 studies every internist should know
Includes bibliographical references and index.
ISBN 978–0–19–934993–7 (alk. paper)
I. Swiger, Kristopher, editor. II. Thomas, Joshua R., editor. III. Hochman, Michael E., editor.
IV. Hochman, Steven, editor. V. Title: 50 studies every internist should know. VI. Series: 50 studies
every doctor should know (Series)
[DNLM: 1. Internal Medicine—methods. 2. Evidence-Based Medicine. 3. Preventive
Medicine—methods. WB 115]
RC46
616—dc23
2014043394

To Shannon, the reason for everything I do.
—KRISTOPHER J. SWIGER, MD

To my wife, Ive Caroline, and children, Jeffrey, Daniel, and Jacob, and to my parents, Jeff and Sharolyn Thomas. Thanks for all of your love and support.
—JOSHUA R. THOMAS, MD, MPH

To the Cambridge Health Alliance Internal Medicine Residency Program, where I learned to practice thoughtful, patient-focused, evidence-based medicine.
—MICHAEL E. HOCHMAN, MD, MPH

To Mom and Hannah.
—STEVEN D. HOCHMAN, MPH

CONTENTS

SECTION 2 Endocrinology

SECTION 3 Hematology and Oncology

SECTION 4 Musculoskeletal Diseases

SECTION 9 Pulmonary and Critical Care Medicine

SECTION 10 Geriatrics and Palliative Care

SECTION 11 Mental Health

PREFACE

This book was written as part of the *50 Studies Every Doctor Should Know* series, with the goal of familiarizing practicing health care providers, trainees, and interested patients with the key studies that form the evidence foundation of adult medicine. The literature upon which we base clinical decisions often feels overwhelming. For the individual trying to make decisions in clinical practice or on the wards, understanding the medical literature may feel both impractical and at times irrelevant. After all, guidelines from professional societies specify best practices in a digestible format. Is that not sufficient?

The trouble is that clinical decision making is often nuanced. For example, recent guidelines recommend a blood pressure target of <150/90 mm Hg for adults ≥60 years of age. But do these recommendations apply to frail, elderly patients? Key studies on hypertension—summarized in this book—provide important insights. These studies have demonstrated a benefit of blood pressure control in the elderly, including those ≥80 years of age. However, these studies excluded patients with major comorbidities like dementia who are at increased risk for medication side effects. Thus, for frail, elderly patients the appropriate management of blood pressure remains uncertain, and optimal care requires consideration of not just the guidelines but also the medical literature as well as patients' individual circumstances. Similarly, major guidelines recommend a mammography screening for all women 50–74 years of age; however, as you will learn in this book, the absolute benefits of such screening are low and there are risks from overdiagnosing cancers that would not otherwise have become clinically apparent. Thus, for a woman who strongly prefers not to undergo screening, it would be quite appropriate to wholeheartedly support her preference, even if it deviates from the guidelines.

In this volume, we have attempted to identify key studies from the field of adult medicine and to present them in an accessible format. Notably, 20 of the studies we selected come directly from the original edition of *50 Studies Every*

Doctor Should Know while 30 are new to this edition. We begin each study summary by identifying the clinical question being addressed; we then summarize the main findings and methodological strengths and weaknesses. We conclude each summary by highlighting the central message and the implications for clinical practice. We also provide a clinical case at the end of each chapter, which provides you with an opportunity to apply the findings in a real life situation.

We hope that you will finish this book not only with a strong understanding of the key studies we discuss but also with a framework for reviewing clinical studies and applying the results to clinical practice. We hope this will enable clinicians and patients alike to make more thoughtful and informed medical decisions.

You may wonder how we selected the studies included here. Based on feedback from the original edition of *50 Studies Every Doctor Should Know*, we used a rigorous selection process in which we surveyed experts in the field of adult medicine, and we used their input to develop our list. Even despite our efforts to use a systematic process to select studies, we suspect that some will quibble with our selections (we certainly quibbled among ourselves as we finalized the list!). Still, we believe the studies we describe cover a wide array of topics in adult medicine and also represent a good starting point for becoming familiar with the medical literature on adults. As examples, we have included a phase I trial of imatinib, which revolutionized not just the treatment of chronic myeloid leukemia, but also the way we think about targeted drug therapy; the Diabetes Control and Complications Trial, which demonstrated the benefits of tight blood sugar control in patients with type 1 diabetes; and a study evaluating the risks and benefits of feeding tube insertion in patients with dementia. As always, we are happy to receive feedback and suggestions for future editions of this book.

From our entire writing team, we hope that you enjoy reading this work and that the medical literature brings to you as much enlightenment as it has brought to us.

Kristopher J. Swiger, MD
Joshua R. Thomas, MD, MPH
Michael E. Hochman, MD, MPH
Steven D. Hochman, MPH

ACKNOWLEDGMENTS

We would like to thank the 40 authors of studies included in this book who graciously reviewed our summaries for accuracy (38 of their names are listed below, and 2 wished to remain anonymous). We very much appreciate the assistance of these authors. Importantly, however, the views expressed in this book do not represent those of the authors acknowledged below, nor do these authors vouch for the accuracy of the information; any mistakes are our own.

- Dr. William C. Knowler, Diabetes Prevention Program Writing Committee: Reduction in the incidence of type 2 diabetes with lifestyle intervention or metformin. *N Engl J Med*. 2002 Feb 7;346(6):393–403.
- Dr. Lawrence Appel, first author: A clinical trial of the effects of dietary patterns on blood pressure. DASH Collaborative Research Group. *N Engl J Med*. 1997;336:1117.
- Dr. Charles H. Hennekens, principal investigator of the Physicians' Health Study Research Group and Chairman of the Steering Committee: Final report on the aspirin component of the ongoing Physicians' Health Study. *N Engl J Med*. 1989 Jul 20;321(3):129–135.
- Dr. Paul M. Ridker, first author: A randomized trial of low-dose aspirin in the primary prevention of cardiovascular disease in women. *N Engl J Med*. 2005 Mar 31;352(13):1293–1304.
- Dr. Rowan T. Chlebowski, member of the Women's Health Initiative Steering Committee: Risks and benefits of estrogen plus progestin in healthy postmenopausal women: principal results from the Women's Health Initiative randomized controlled trial. *JAMA*. 2002 Jul 17;288(3):321–333.
- Dr. Fritz H. Schröder, first author: Prostate-cancer mortality at 11 years of follow-up. *N Engl J Med*. 2012 Mar 15;366(11):981–990.

- Dr. Denise Alberle, of the National Lung Screening Trial Research Team: Reduced lung-cancer mortality with low-dose computed tomographic screening. *N Engl J Med.* 2011;365(5):395–409.
- Ms. Patricia Cleary, principal investigator of the Diabetes Control and Complications Trial Research Group: The effect of intensive treatment of diabetes on the development and progression of long-term complications in insulin-dependent diabetes mellitus. The Diabetes Control and Complications Trial Research Group. *N Engl J Med.* 1993;329:977.
- Dr. William Cushman, ACCORD Study investigator: Effects of intensive blood-pressure control in type 2 diabetes mellitus. *N Engl J Med.* 2010;362:1575.
- Dr. Brian Druker, first author: Efficacy and safety of a specific inhibitor of the BCR-ABL tyrosine kinase in chronic myeloid leukemia. *N Engl J Med.* 2001;344:1031.
- Dr. Jeffrey (Jerry) G. Jarvik, first author: Rapid magnetic resonance imaging vs. radiographs for patients with low back pain: a randomized controlled trial. *JAMA.* 2003;289(21):2810–2818.
- Drs. Catriona Grigor and Duncan Porter, first and senior authors: Effect of a treatment strategy of tight control for rheumatoid arthritis (the TICORA study): a single-blind randomised controlled trial. *Lancet.* 2004 Jul 17–23;364(9430);263–269.
- Dr. Keith Wheatley, ASTRAL investigator: Revascularization versus medical therapy for renal-artery stenosis. *N Engl J Med.* 2009;361:1953.
- Dr. Juan Carlos Garcia-Pagan, Early TIPS Corporative Study Group: Early use of TIPS in patients with cirrhosis and variceal bleeding. *N Engl J Med.* 2010 June 24;362(25):2370–2379.
- Dr. Gregory Moran, EMERGEncy ID Net Study Group: Methicillin-resistant *S. aureus* infections among patients in the emergency department. *N Engl J Med.* 2006;355:666–674.
- Dr. Paul M. Ridker, principal investigator, trial chair, and first author: Rosuvastatin to prevent vascular events in men and women with elevated C-reactive protein. *N Engl J Med.* 2008 Nov 20;359(21):2195–2207.
- Dr. Terje Pedersen, 4S Study investigator: Randomised trial of cholesterol lowering in 4,444 patients with coronary heart disease: the Scandinavian Simvastatin Survival Study (4S). *Lancet.* 1994;344:1383.
- Dr. William C. Cushman, member of the ALLHAT Group Steering Committee: Major outcomes in high-risk hypertensive patients

randomized to angiotensin-converting enzyme inhibitor or calcium channel blocker vs diuretic: the antihypertensive and lipid-lowering treatment to prevent heart attack trial (ALLHAT). *JAMA*. 2002 Dec 18;288(23):2981–2997.

- Dr. Brian Olshanksy, AFFIRM investigator: A comparison of rate control and rhythm control in patients with atrial fibrillation. *N Engl J Med*. 2002 Dec 5;347(23):1825–1833.
- Dr. William E. Boden, cochair for the COURAGE Trial Research Group, and first author: Optimal medical therapy with or without PCI for stable coronary disease. *N Engl J Med*. 2007 Apr 12;356(15):1503–1516.
- Dr. Keith Fox, Randomized Intervention Trial of Unstable Angina Investigators: Interventional versus conservative treatment for patients with unstable angina or non-ST-elevation myocardial infarction: the British Heart Foundation RITA 3 randomized trial. *Lancet* 2002;360:743–751.
- Dr. Arthur Moss, Multicenter Automatic Defibrillator Implantation Trial II investigator: Prophylactic implantation of a defibrillator in patients with myocardial infarction and reduced ejection fraction. *N Engl J Med*. 2002;346:877.
- Dr. Anne L. Taylor, chair of the A-HeFT Steering Committee and first author: Combination of isosorbidedinitrate and hydralazine in blacks with heart failure. *N Engl J Med*. 2004 Nov 11;351(20):2049–2056.
- Dr. Holger Thiele, IABP-SHOCK II Study investigator: Intraaortic balloon support for myocardial infarction with cardiogenic shock. *N Engl J Med*. 2012;367:1287.
- Dr. Simon Finfer, NICE-SUGAR Study investigator: Intensive versus conventional glucose control in critically ill patients. *NEJM*. 2009;360(13):1283–1297.
- Dr. Paul C. Hébert, first author: A multicenter, randomized, controlled clinical trial of transfusion requirements in critical care. *N Engl J Med*. 1999 Feb 11;340(6):409–417.
- Dr. Laurent Brochard, first author: Noninvasive ventilation for acute exacerbations of chronic obstructive pulmonary disease. *N Engl J Med*. 1995 Sep 28;333(13):817–822.
- Dr. Roy Brower, ARDS Network: Ventilation with lower tidal volumes as compared with traditional tidal volumes for ALI and ARDS. *N Engl J Med*. 2000;342:1301–1308.
- Dr. Emanuel Rivers, first author: Early goal-directed therapy in the treatment of severe sepsis and septic shock. *N Engl J Med*. 2001 Nov 8;345(19):1368–1377.

- Dr. Daniel De Backer, SOAP II investigator: Comparison of dopamine and norepinephrine in the treatment of shock. *N Engl J Med.* 2010 Mar 4;362(9):779–789.
- Dr. John Kress, first author: Daily interruption of sedative infusions in critically ill patients undergoing mechanical ventilation. *N Engl J Med.* 2000;342:1471.
- Dr. Andres Esteban, first author: A comparison of four methods of weaning patients from mechanical ventilation. Spanish Lung Failure Collaborative Group. *N Engl J Med.* 1995;332:345.
- Dr. Charles M. Morin, first author: Behavioral and pharmacological therapies for late-life insomnia: a randomized controlled trial. *JAMA.* 1999;281(11):991–999.
- Dr. Nigel Beckett, HYVET Study Group: Treatment of hypertension in patients 80 years of age and older. *New Eng J Med.* 2008;358:1887–1898.
- Dr. Joan Teno, first author: Does feeding tube insertion and its timing improve survival? *J Am Geriatr Soc.* 2012;60:1918.
- Dr. Jennifer S. Temel, first author: Early palliative care for patients with metastatic non-small-cell lung cancer. *N Engl J Med.* 2010 Aug 19;363(8):733–742.
- Dr. Herbert C. Schulberg, first author: Treating major depression in primary care practice. *Arch Gen Psychiatry.* 1996;53:913–919.
- Dr. Richard Saitz, first author: Individualized treatment for alcohol withdrawal: a randomized double-blind controlled trial. *JAMA.* 1994;272:519.

CONTRIBUTORS

Adel Boueiz, MD
Fellow, Pulmonary and Critical
    Care Medicine
Department of Medicine
Massachusetts General Hospital
Boston, Massachusetts

William Butron, MD
Resident, Internal Medicine
    and Pediatrics
Department of Internal Medicine
    and Pediatrics
University of Oklahoma
Tulsa, Oklahoma

Lavanya Kondapalli, MD
Fellow, Cardio-Oncology
Division of Cardiovascular Medicine
Hospital of the University of
    Pennsylvania
Philadelphia, Pennsylvania

Thomas Kriley, MD
North Colorado Family Medicine
Greeley, Colorado

Vimal Ramjee, MD
Fellow, Cardiovascular Disease
Division of Cardiovascular Medicine
University of Pennsylvania
Philadelphia, Pennsylvania

Laalitha Surapaneni, MBBS, MPH
Bloomberg School of Public Health
Johns Hopkins University School of
    Medicine
Baltimore, Maryland

Kathryn White, DO
Resident, Internal Medicine
Department of Internal Medicine
University of Oklahoma
Tulsa, Oklahoma

SECTION 1

Preventive Medicine

1

Preventing Diabetes

The Diabetes Prevention Program

MICHAEL E. HOCHMAN

> Our study showed that treatment with metformin and modification of lifestyle were two highly effective means of delaying or preventing type 2 diabetes. The lifestyle intervention was particularly effective, with one case of diabetes prevented per seven persons treated for three years.
> —THE DIABETES PREVENTION PROGRAM RESEARCH GROUP[1]

Research Question: Can the onset of type 2 diabetes be prevented or delayed with metformin and/or lifestyle modifications?[1]

Funding: The National Institutes of Health, the Indian Health Service, the Centers for Disease Control and Prevention, the General Clinical Research Center Program, the American Diabetes Association, Bristol-Myers Squibb, and Parke-Davis Pharmaceuticals.

Year Study Began: 1996

Year Study Published: 2002

Study Location: 27 clinical centers in the United States.

Who Was Studied: Adults $\geq$25 years old with a body mass index (BMI) $\geq$24 kg/m^2, a fasting plasma glucose of 95–125 mg/dL, and a plasma glucose of 140–199 mg/dL 2 hours after a 75-g oral glucose load.

Who Was Excluded: People with diagnosed diabetes, those taking medications known to alter glucose tolerance, and those with serious illnesses that could reduce life expectancy or interfere with the ability to participate in the trial.

How Many Participants: 3,234

Study Overview: See Figure 1.1 for a summary of the trial's design.

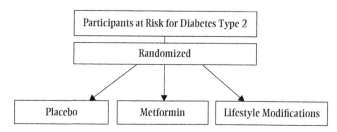

Figure 1.1 Summary of the Study Design.

Study Interventions: Participants in the placebo group received standard lifestyle recommendations. Participants in the metformin group received standard lifestyle recommendations along with metformin 850 mg twice daily. Participants in the lifestyle group were given an intensive lifestyle modification program taught by case managers on a one-to-one basis with the goal of achieving and maintaining a 7% or greater reduction in body weight, improvements in dietary intake, and physical activity of at least 150 minutes per week. The lifestyle modification program was taught during 16 sessions over a 24-week period, and reinforced with individual (usually monthly) and group sessions after that.

Follow-Up: Mean of 2.8 years.

Endpoint: Primary outcome: Diabetes, as defined by either a fasting glucose ≥126 mg/dL or a glucose ≥200 2 hours after a 75-g oral glucose load on two separate occasions.

RESULTS

- The average participant in the lifestyle group lost 5.6 kg during the study period versus 2.1 kg in the metformin group and 0.1 kg in the placebo group ($P < 0.001$).

- Participants in the lifestyle group reported significantly more physical activity than those in the metformin and placebo groups, and at the final study visit 58% reported at least 150 minutes per week of physical activity.
- Participants in the metformin group had approximately six times the rate of gastrointestinal symptoms as participants in the lifestyle group, while the rate of musculoskeletal symptoms was approximately 1.2 times higher among participants in the lifestyle group compared with those in the metformin group.
- Participants in the lifestyle group had the lowest incidence of diabetes during the study (see Table 1.1).

Table 1.1. SUMMARY OF KEY FINDINGS

	Placebo	Metformin	Lifestyle Modifications
Estimated Cumulative Incidence of Diabetes at 3 Years	28.9%[a]	21.7%[a]	14.4%[a]

[a] Differences all statistically significant.

Criticisms and Limitations: The participants assigned to the lifestyle group achieved an impressive reduction in weight as well as impressive improvements in dietary and exercise patterns. This suggests that study participants were highly motivated individuals. Such successes might not be possible in other populations. In addition, the trial did not assess whether either the lifestyle intervention or metformin led to a reduction in hard clinical endpoints, such as diabetes-related microvascular disease.

Other Relevant Studies and Information:

- Several other studies have demonstrated that lifestyle interventions can delay the development of diabetes in at-risk patients.[2]
- A recently published 10-year follow-up evaluation of participants in the Diabetes Prevention Program showed that the cumulative incidence of diabetes remained 34% lower in the lifestyle group and 18% lower in the metformin group compared with the placebo group.[3]
- A cost-effectiveness analysis demonstrated that over 10 years, the lifestyle intervention used in the Diabetes Prevention Program was cost-effective and metformin was marginally cost-saving compared with placebo.[4-7]

- The American Diabetes Association recommends lifestyle efforts as the primary method for preventing diabetes in those with impaired glucose tolerance, impaired fasting glucose, and/or a hemoglobin A1c of 5.7–6.4%. In certain high-risk individuals, metformin may also be considered, however.[8]

Summary and Implications: To prevent one case of diabetes over 3 years, approximately seven people must be treated with a lifestyle intervention program or approximately 14 must be treated with metformin. Lifestyle modifications are, therefore, the preferred method for preventing or delaying the onset of diabetes.

CLINICAL CASE: PREVENTING DIABETES

Case History:

A 54-year-old woman is found to have prediabetes with a fasting plasma glucose of 116 on two separate occasions. She is overweight, with a BMI of 29, and reports only very limited physical activity.

As this woman's doctor, you recommend that she begin a weight-loss and exercise program to reduce her risk for developing diabetes. But she is hesitant and tells you she is too busy to make lifestyle changes. In addition, "none of this lifestyle stuff works anyway."

Based on the results of the Diabetes Prevention Program, what can you tell your patient about the potential impact of lifestyle changes for preventing diabetes?

Suggested Answer:

The Diabetes Prevention Program unequivocally demonstrated that lifestyle modifications—more so than medications—can reduce the risk of developing diabetes. Thus, you can tell your patient that there is good evidence from a well-designed study that lifestyle changes can work.

Since this woman is busy and may not have the time to participate in an intensive program, as the study participants in the Diabetes Prevention Program did, you might give her some simple recommendations she can follow on her own, for example, walking for 30 minutes a day. You might also give her manageable goals, for example, a 5- to 10-pound weight loss at her next visit with you in 3 months.

References

1. Diabetes Prevention Program Research Group. Reduction in the incidence of type 2 diabetes with lifestyle intervention or metformin. *N Engl J Med.* 2002;346(6):393–403.
2. Tuomilehto J et al. Prevention of type 2 diabetes mellitus by changes in lifestyle among subjects with impaired glucose tolerance. *N Engl J Med.* 2001;344(18):1343.
3. Diabetes Prevention Program Research Group. 10-year follow-up of diabetes incidence and weight loss in the Diabetes Prevention Program outcomes study. *Lancet.* 2009;374(9702):1677–1686.
4. Diabetes Prevention Program Research Group. The 10-year cost-effectiveness of lifestyle intervention or metformin for diabetes prevention: an intent-to-treat analysis of the DPP/DPPOS. *Diabetes Care.* 2012;35(4):723–730.
5. Li G et al. The long-term effect of lifestyle interventions to prevent diabetes in the China Da Qing Diabetes Prevention Study: a 20-year follow-up study. *Lancet.* 2008;371(9626):1783.
6. Saito T et al. Lifestyle modification and prevention of type 2 diabetes in overweight Japanese with impaired fasting glucose levels: a randomized controlled trial. *Arch Intern Med.* 2011;171(15):1352.
7. Davey Smith G et al. Incidence of type 2 diabetes in the randomized multiple risk factor intervention trial. *Ann Intern Med.* 2005;142(5):313.
8. American Diabetes Association. Standards of medical care in diabetes—2014. *Diabetes Care.* 2014;37(Suppl 1):S14.

2

Dietary Approaches to Stop Hypertension (DASH)

STEVEN D. HOCHMAN

> A diet rich in fruits, vegetables, and low-fat dairy foods . . . can substantially lower blood pressure.
>
> —APPEL ET AL.[1]

Research Question: Can modification of dietary patterns lower blood pressure in patients with prehypertension and/or stage I hypertension?[1]

Funding: The National Heart, Lung, and Blood Institute, and the Office of Research on Minority Health.

Year Study Began: 1994

Year Study Published: 1997

Study Location: Multiple sites in the United States.

Who Was Studied: Adults ≥22 years of age with a diastolic blood pressure between 80 and 95 mm Hg and a systolic blood pressure ≤160 mm Hg who were not taking any antihypertensive medications.

Who Was Excluded: Patients with a body mass index (BMI) >35, those with poorly controlled diabetes mellitus or dyslipidemia, those with a cardiovascular event in the previous 6 months, renal insufficiency, or a chronic disease that could interfere with participation. Also excluded were patients taking medications affecting blood pressure, those with heavy alcohol use, and those unwilling or unable to discontinue supplements or antacids containing magnesium or calcium.

How Many Patients: 459

Study Overview: See Figure 2.1 for a summary of the study's design.

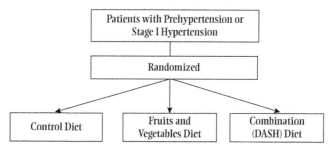

Figure 2.1 Summary of the Study Design.

Study Intervention: Participants were randomized to one of three diets:

- Control diet: Potassium, magnesium, and calcium levels at the 25th percentile of US consumption, and protein, carbohydrates, fats, and fiber at average US consumption ("typical American diet").
- Fruits and vegetables diet: Potassium and magnesium levels at the 75th percentile of US consumption and high content of fiber, fruits, and vegetables.
- Combination (DASH) diet: High content of fiber, fruits, and vegetables (fruits and vegetables diet) plus high in protein and low-fat dairy; also low in saturated and total fat.

All diets were low in sodium (3,000 mg/day).

Participants followed their prescribed diets for 8 weeks. Each day, participants ate one meal at the study center and were provided meals to be eaten offsite. Participants were instructed to avoid nonstudy food and to limit caffeinated beverages to fewer than three per day and alcoholic beverages to fewer than two per day. The total calories per day were adjusted for the participants to maintain a stable weight.

Follow-Up: 8 weeks.

Endpoints: Primary outcome: Change in diastolic blood pressure. Secondary outcome: Change in systolic blood pressure.

RESULTS

- Baseline characteristics were similar between the groups with a mean age of 44 years and mean blood pressure of 132/85; 51% of participants were female and 59% were black.
- Adherence to the prescribed diets was high for all three groups.
- The mean decrease in blood pressure was greater in the combination (DASH) diet compared to the fruits and vegetables diet and the control diet (Table 2.1).
- The mean decrease in blood pressure was most pronounced among patients enrolled with a diagnosis of hypertension (Table 2.1) and was consistent across several subgroups, including those stratified by gender and minority status.
- The mean decrease in systolic blood pressure was greater in the fruits and vegetables diet compared to the control diet (-2.8 mm Hg, $P < 0.001$).

Table 2.1. SUMMARY OF KEY FINDINGS

	DASH Diet versus Control Diet	P Value	DASH Diet versus Fruits and Vegetables Diet	P Value
Change in Systolic Blood Pressure	-5.5 mm Hg	<0.001	-2.7 mm Hg	0.001
Among Patients with Hypertension	-11.4 mm Hg	<0.001	-4.1 mm Hg	0.04
Change in Diastolic Blood Pressure	-3.0 mm Hg	<0.001	-1.9 mm Hg	0.002
Among Patients with Hypertension	-5.5 mm Hg	<0.001	-2.6 mm Hg	0.03

Criticisms and Limitations: This trial was an efficacy study in which participants received all of the food that they ate. It is likely that dietary compliance would be lower outside of an experimental setting, and thus the effects of these dietary changes would likely be considerably lower. Reassuringly, however, favorable results were also obtained in a study of the DASH diet in which participants were not provided with meals during the study period (see "Other Relevant Studies and Information").

In addition, because the study tested the effects of whole dietary patterns, it is not clear from this study which elements of the study diet were responsible for the observed reductions in blood pressure.

Other Relevant Studies and Information:

- Additional studies of the DASH diet compared to control diets have demonstrated similar results. In another feeding study by the same research group, the DASH diet and sodium reduction, alone and combined, lowered blood pressure.[2]
- The PREMIER trial demonstrated significant blood pressure reduction among patients who received a behavioral intervention that included the DASH diet along with other lifestyle factors that lower blood pressure (weight loss, increased physical activity, and sodium reduction); unlike the original DASH trial, participants in PREMIER received counseling as opposed to prepared food from the investigators.[3]

Summary and Implications: The results of this trial demonstrate that modification of diet can have powerful effects on blood pressure, especially for persons with hypertension. The DASH diet confers an average reduction of systolic blood pressure by 5.5 mm Hg and of diastolic blood pressure by 3.0 mm Hg relative to a diet that many people typically eat, and an average reduction of 2.7 mm Hg/1.9 mm Hg relative to a diet high in fruits and vegetables. Though compliance with the DASH diet may be challenging in real-world settings, these results provide strong evidence that dietary modifications can lower blood pressure among patients with prehypertension and stage I hypertension.

CLINICAL CASE: DASH DIET

Case History:
A 34-year-old man presents to the clinic for a routine follow-up. He was last seen 2 years ago, at which time his blood pressure was 132/86. He is in good health and reports that he jogs for 30 minutes three to four times per week. He lives alone and reports that he eats fast food multiple times per week and prefers meat and potatoes when he cooks for himself. He does not add salt to his food, but he reports eating prepackaged soups and potato chips that he knows are high in sodium. His vital signs in the clinic today are notable for a blood pressure of 144/94 and a heart rate of 72. His BMI is 28.

Based on the results of this trial, how would you manage this patient's blood pressure?

Suggested Answer:

The patient's blood pressure is elevated today. Although a second measurement would be necessary to make the diagnosis of hypertension, his blood pressure was already in the prehypertensive range prior to today's visit, and it is likely that he would benefit from lifestyle changes aimed at lowering his blood pressure. Specifically, he might increase his physical activity, lose weight, further reduce sodium intake, and make dietary changes consistent with those in the DASH diet (rich in fruits, vegetables, and low-fat dairy, and low in saturated fat and cholesterol). You might also refer him to a nutritionist or health educator to provide detailed teaching on these dietary changes.

The patient should also be instructed to monitor his blood pressure regularly (perhaps he could track his blood pressure at home with a cuff). If his blood pressure remains in the hypertensive range despite lifestyle modifications, pharmacologic therapy may ultimately be needed.

References

1. Appel LJ et al. A clinical trial of the effects of dietary patterns on blood pressure. DASH Collaborative Research Group. *N Engl J Med*. 1997;336:1117.
2. Sacks FM et al. Effects on blood pressure of reduced dietary sodium and the Dietary Approaches to Stop Hypertension (DASH) diet. DASH-Sodium Collaborative Research Group. *N Engl J Med*. 2001;344:3.
3. Appel LJ et al. Effects of comprehensive lifestyle modification on blood pressure control: main results of the PREMIER clinical trial. *JAMA*. 2003;289:2083.

3

Aspirin for the Primary Prevention of Cardiovascular Disease

The Physicians' Health Study and the Women's Health Study

MICHAEL E. HOCHMAN

[The Physicians' Health Study] demonstrates a conclusive reduction in the risk of myocardial infarction [in men], but the evidence concerning stroke and total cardiovascular deaths remains inconclusive . . . as expected, [aspirin led to] increased risks of upper gastrointestinal ulcers and bleeding problems.

—THE PHYSICIANS' HEALTH STUDY RESEARCH GROUP[1]

[In the Women's Health Study] aspirin lowered the risk of stroke without affecting the risk of myocardial infarction or death from cardiovascular causes . . . as expected, the frequency of side effects related to bleeding and ulcers was increased.

—RIDKER ET AL.[2]

Research Question: Is aspirin effective for the prevention of cardiovascular disease in apparently healthy adults?[1,2]

Funding: The Physicians' Health Study was sponsored by the National Institutes of Health, and the Women's Health Study was sponsored by the National Heart, Lung, and Blood Institute and the National Cancer Institute.

Year Study Began: 1982 (Physicians' Health Study) and 1992 (Women's Health Study)

Year Study Published: 1989 (Physicians' Health Study) and 2005 (Women's Health Study)

Study Location: The Physicians' Health Study was open to apparently healthy male physicians throughout the United States who were mailed invitations to participate. The Women's Health Study was open to apparently healthy female health professionals throughout the United States who were mailed invitations to participate.

Who Was Studied: The Physicians' Health Study included apparently healthy male physicians 40–84, while the Women's Health Study included apparently healthy female health professionals ≥45.

Who Was Excluded: Patients were excluded from both trials if they had existing cardiovascular disease, cancer, other chronic medical problems, or if they were currently taking aspirin or nonsteroidal anti-inflammatory agents. Both trials included a run-in period to identify patients unlikely to be compliant with the study protocol, and these patients were excluded before randomization.

How Many Patients: The Physicians' Health Study included 22,071 men, while the Women's Health Study included 39,876 women.

Study Overview: See Figure 3.1 for a summary of the trials' design.

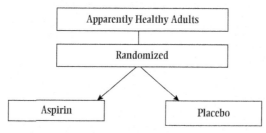

Figure 3.1 Summary of the Study Design.

Study Intervention: In the Physicians' Health Study, patients in the aspirin group received aspirin 325 mg on alternate days while in the Women's Health Study patients in the aspirin group received aspirin 100 mg on alternate days. In both trials, patients in the control group received a placebo pill on alternate days.

Follow-Up: Approximately 5 years for the Physicians' Health Study and approximately 10 years for the Women's Health Study.

Endpoints: Myocardial infarction, stroke, cardiovascular mortality, and hemorrhagic side effects.

RESULTS

- In both trials, aspirin led to a small reduction in cardiovascular events but an increase in bleeding events (see Tables 3.1 and 3.2).
- In both trials, aspirin was most beneficial among older patients (men ≥50 and women ≥65).

Table 3.1. SUMMARY OF THE PHYSICIANS' HEALTH STUDY'S KEY FINDINGS

Outcome	Aspirin Group	Placebo Group	P Value
Myocardial Infarction	1.3%	2.2%	<0.00001
Stroke	1.1%	0.9%	0.15
Cardiovascular Mortality	0.7%	0.8%	0.87
Gastrointestinal Ulcers	1.5%	1.3%	0.08
Bleeding Requiring Transfusion	0.4%	0.3%	0.02

Table 3.2. SUMMARY OF THE WOMEN'S HEALTH STUDY'S KEY FINDINGS

Outcome	Aspirin Group	Placebo Group	P Value
Cardiovascular Events[a]	2.4%	2.6%	0.13
Stroke	1.1%	1.3%	0.04
Myocardial Infarction	1.0%	1.0%	0.83
Cardiovascular Mortality	0.6%	0.6%	0.68
Gastrointestinal Bleeding	4.6%	3.8%	<0.001

[a] Includes myocardial infarction, stroke, and death from cardiovascular causes.

Criticisms and Limitations: In the Physicians' Health Study, aspirin 325 mg was given on alternate days while in the Women's Health Study aspirin 100 mg was given on alternate days. In clinical practice, however, most patients receive aspirin 81 mg daily (data concerning the optimal ASA dose are sparse).

Both of these trials are limited in generalizability. Both included patients of high socioeconomic status. In addition, patients found to be noncompliant during a run-in period were excluded. Patients in the general population are likely to be less compliant with therapy, and therefore the benefits of aspirin observed in real-world settings may be lower.

Other Relevant Studies and Information:

- Other trials of aspirin for cardiovascular disease prevention have also suggested that aspirin reduces the risk of cardiovascular events while increasing bleeding risk.[3]
- Some data have suggested that aspirin decreases the incidence of colorectal cancer, but the benefits appear modest and more data are needed to confirm this conclusion.[4]
- Whether aspirin has a differential effect on men and women is unclear: one meta-analysis suggested that in men aspirin may preferentially prevent myocardial infarctions while in women aspirin may preferentially prevent strokes.[5] Other experts believe this conclusion is premature, however.[6]
- Aspirin is also effective in preventing cardiovascular events in high-risk patients with vascular disease,[7] and the absolute benefits are greater among these patients.

The American Heart Association recommends daily aspirin for apparently healthy men and women whose 10-year risk of a first event exceeds 10%, while the US Preventive Services Task Force recommends low-dose (e.g., 75 mg) daily aspirin for primary cardiovascular prevention in the following circumstances:

- In women 55–79 when the reduction in ischemic stroke risk is greater than the increase in gastrointestinal hemorrhage risk (e.g., a woman with a high stroke risk but low bleeding risk would be a good candidate while a woman with a high bleeding risk but low stroke risk would not be).
- In men 45–79 when the reduction in the risk of myocardial infarction is greater than the increase in gastrointestinal hemorrhage risk (e.g., a man with a high risk of myocardial infarction but low bleeding risk would be a good candidate while a man with a high bleeding risk but low risk of myocardial infarction would not be).

Summary and Implications: In apparently healthy men and women, aspirin leads to a small reduction in the risk of cardiovascular disease while increasing bleeding risk. In men, aspirin may preferentially prevent myocardial infarctions, while in women aspirin may preferentially prevent strokes, though this conclusion is uncertain. Aspirin can be considered for primary cardiovascular prevention in both men and women with cardiovascular risk factors when the risk of gastrointestinal hemorrhage is low.

CLINICAL CASE: ASPIRIN FOR THE PRIMARY PREVENTION OF CARDIOVASCULAR DISEASE

Case History:

A 60-year-old woman with a history of hypertension, hyperlipidemia, liver cirrhosis, esophageal varices, and recurrent gastrointestinal bleeding asks whether she should receive aspirin to reduce her risk of cardiovascular disease. Based on the results of the Women's Health Study, what would you recommend?

Suggested Answer:

The Women's Health Study demonstrated that, in female health professionals ≥45, daily aspirin leads to a small but detectable reduction in the risk of cardiovascular disease while increasing bleeding risk. The US Preventive Services Task Force recommends low-dose daily aspirin in women 55–79 when the reduction in cardiovascular risk is judged to be greater than the increase in risk of gastrointestinal hemorrhage.

The patient in this vignette has risk factors for cardiovascular disease and therefore might be a candidate for aspirin. However, she has numerous risk factors for gastrointestinal bleeding, making aspirin therapy risky. Overall, the risks of aspirin likely outweigh the benefits in this patient.

References

1. The Physicians' Health Study Research Group. Final report on the aspirin component of the ongoing Physicians' Health Study. *N Engl J Med.* 1989;321(3):129–135.
2. Ridker PM et al. A randomized trial of low-dose aspirin in the primary prevention of cardiovascular disease in women. *N Engl J Med.* 2005;352(13):1293–1304.
3. Antithrombotic Trialists' (ATT) Collaboration. Aspirin in the primary and secondary prevention of vascular disease: collaborative meta-analysis of individual participant data from randomised trials. *Lancet.* 2009;373(9678):1849.
4. Dubé C et al. The use of aspirin for primary prevention of colorectal cancer: a systematic review prepared for the U.S. Preventive Services Task Force. *Ann Intern Med.* 2007;146(5):365.

5. Berger JS et al. Aspirin for the primary prevention of cardiovascular events in women and men: a sex-specific meta-analysis of randomized controlled trials. *JAMA*. 2006;295(3):306.

6. Hennekens CH et al. Sex-related differences in response to aspirin in cardiovascular disease: an untested hypothesis. *Nat Clin Pract Cardiovasc Med*. 2006;3:4–5.

7. Berger JS et al. Low-dose aspirin in patients with stable cardiovascular disease: a meta-analysis. *Am J Med*. 2008;121(1):43.

4

Postmenopausal Hormone Therapy

The Women's Health Initiative (WHI)

MICHAEL E. HOCHMAN

> The [Women's Health Initiative] provides an important health answer
> for generations of healthy postmenopausal women to come—do not
> use estrogen/progestin to prevent chronic disease.
>
> —FLETCHER AND COLDITZ[1]

Research Question: Should postmenopausal women take combined hormone
therapy for the prevention of cardiovascular disease and fractures?[2]

Funding: The National Heart, Lung, and Blood Institute.

Year Study Began: 1993

Year Study Published: 2002

Study Location: 40 clinical centers throughout the United States.

Who Was Studied: Postmenopausal women 50–79 years of age.

Who Was Excluded: Patients with a prior hysterectomy, those with another
serious medical condition associated with a life expectancy of less than 3 years,
or those with a history of cancer.

How Many Patients: 16,608

Study Overview: See Figure 4.1 for a summary of the WHI's design.

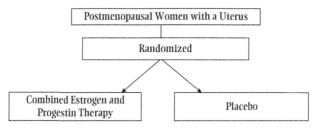

Figure 4.1 Summary of the Study Design.

Study Intervention: Patients in the combined hormone therapy group received one tablet of conjugated equine estrogen 0.625 mg and medroxyprogesterone acetate 2.5 mg daily. Patients in the control group received a placebo tablet.

Follow-Up: Mean of 5.6 years (8.5 years of therapy were planned, but the intervention was stopped early because initial results showed that the health risks exceeded the benefits). (The follow-up was originally reported as 5.2 years but more accurately was 5.6 years, according to Dr. Rowan Chlebowski, a member of the Women's Health Initiative's Steering Committee.)

Endpoints: Primary outcomes: Coronary heart disease (nonfatal or fatal myocardial infarction) and invasive breast cancer. Other major outcomes: Stroke, pulmonary embolism, hip fracture, death, and a global index summarizing the risks and benefits of combined hormone therapy.

RESULTS

- Combined hormone therapy led to an increase in cardiovascular disease and breast cancer but a reduction in hip fractures (see Table 4.1).
- The global index score summarizing the risks and benefits of combined hormone therapy suggested a small overall harm from combined hormone therapy.

Table 4.1. SUMMARY OF KEY FINDINGS

Outcome	Combined Hormone Therapy Group[a]	Placebo Group[a]	Statistically Significant?[b]
Myocardial Infarctions	0.37%	0.30%	borderline
Stroke	0.29%	0.21%	yes
Venous Thromboembolic Disease	0.34%	0.16%	yes
Invasive Breast Cancer	0.38%	0.30%	borderline
Hip Fracture	0.10%	0.15%	yes
Mortality	0.52%	0.53%	no

[a] Percentages represent average annualized rates, that is, the percentage of people who experienced each outcome per year.
[b] Exact *P* values not reported.

Criticisms and Limitations: The trial only tested one dose and one formulation of combined hormone therapy. It is possible that the risks and benefits are different when lower doses or different formulations of estrogens and progestins are used.

Other Relevant Studies and Information:

- Other studies evaluating combined hormone therapy are generally consistent with those of the WHI.[3]
- Observational studies (case control and cohort studies) prior to the WHI suggested that combined hormone therapy decreased the risk of cardiovascular disease.[4,5] It is now believed that these studies came to erroneous conclusions because women taking combined hormone therapy tended to be healthier than those who weren't, making it appear as though combined hormone therapy reduced the risk of cardiovascular disease.
- The HERS trial showed that, among women with existing heart disease, there was a higher rate of venous thromboembolism among women who took combined hormone therapy.[6]
- The WHI included a separate evaluation of unopposed estrogen therapy (without a progestin) in women with prior hysterectomies. This study suggested an increased rate of stroke among users of estrogen therapy, but the rates of heart attacks and breast cancer were similar in the estrogen and placebo groups.[7]

- An 11-year follow-up evaluation of patients in the WHI showed that breast cancers among women who took combined hormone therapy were more likely to be advanced stage and that breast cancer mortality rates were higher compared to women in the placebo group.[8]
- Recent data have suggested that combined hormone therapy may be less harmful—or even beneficial—if initiated shortly after the onset of menopause,[9,10]; however, these findings are preliminary and controversial.
- Guidelines from the US Preventive Services Task Force recommend against the use of hormone therapy for disease prevention, though hormone therapy may be appropriate for women to manage symptoms of menopause.[11]

Summary and Implications: The WHI showed that the risks (cardiovascular disease, thromboembolic disease, and breast cancer) of combined hormone therapy outweigh the benefits (a reduction in fractures). Since the absolute risks are small, combined hormone therapy remains an option for the management of postmenopausal symptoms; however, combined hormone therapy should only be used when other therapies have failed. The WHI also contains an important lesson for the medical community: except in unusual circumstances, randomized trials—not case-control or cohort studies—are needed before new therapies become the standard of care.

CLINICAL CASE: POSTMENOPAUSAL HORMONE THERAPY

Case History:
A 52-year-old woman with an intact uterus reports persistent and bothersome hot flashes and vaginal dryness since undergoing menopause 1 year ago. The symptoms have not responded to relaxation techniques, and she asks about the possibility of starting hormone therapy to control the symptoms.

Based on the results of the Women's Health Initiative study, what can you tell her about the risks of hormone therapy?

Suggested Answer:
The Women's Health Initiative suggested that long-term (greater than 5 years) combined estrogen and progestin therapy is associated with increased rates of myocardial infarction, stroke, venous thromboembolism, and breast cancer, and a reduced rate of hip fractures. However, given that the absolute increase in disease rates is small, short-term (ideally 2 to 3 years) hormone therapy is

an acceptable treatment for bothersome menopausal symptoms that do not respond to other therapies.

Women in the Women's Health Initiative received hormone therapy for a mean of 5.6 years; the risks of short-term therapy are likely to be lower. In addition, women in the study received conjugated equine estrogen 0.625 mg and medroxyprogesterone acetate 2.5 mg daily. Some experts believe that hormone preparations with lower doses may be safer although there are no data to support these claims. Finally, recent data suggest that combined hormone therapy may be safer when initiated in younger women shortly after menopause.

References

1. Fletcher SW, Colditz GA. Failure of estrogen plus progestin therapy for prevention. *JAMA*. 2002;288:366–368.
2. The Women's Health Initiative Investigators. Risks and benefits of estrogen plus progestin in healthy postmenopausal women: principal results from the Women's Health Initiative randomized controlled trial. *JAMA*. 2002;288(3):321–333.
3. Nelson HD et al. Menopausal hormone therapy for the primary prevention of chronic conditions: a systematic review to update the U.S. Preventive Services Task Force recommendations. *Ann Intern Med*. 2012;157(2):104.
4. Stampfer M, Colditz G. Estrogen replacement therapy and coronary heart disease: a quantitative assessment of the epidemiologic evidence. *Prev Med*. 1991;20:47–63.
5. Grady D et al. Combined hormone therapy to prevent disease and prolong life in postmenopausal women. *Ann Intern Med*. 1992;117:1016–1037.
6. Hulley S et al. Noncardiovascular disease outcomes during 6.8 years of combined hormone therapy: Heart and Estrogen/progestin Replacement Study follow-up (HERS II). *JAMA*. 2002;288(1):58–66.
7. Anderson GL et al. Effects of conjugated equine estrogen in postmenopausal women with hysterectomy: the Women's Health Initiative randomized controlled trial. *JAMA*. 2004;291(14):1701–1712.
8. Chlebowski RT et al. Estrogen plus progestin and breast cancer incidence and mortality in postmenopausal women. *JAMA*. 2010;304(15):1684–1692.
9. Salpeter SR et al. Brief report: Coronary heart disease events associated with hormone therapy in younger and older women: a meta-analysis. *J Gen Intern Med*. 2006;21(4):363.
10. Schierbeck LL et al. Effect of hormone replacement therapy on cardiovascular events in recently postmenopausal women: randomised trial. *BMJ*. 2012;345:e6409.
11. Moyer VA, US Preventive Services Task Force. Menopausal hormone therapy for the primary prevention of chronic conditions: U.S. Preventive Services Task Force recommendation statement. *Ann Intern Med*. 2013;158(1):47.

5

The Cochrane Review of Screening Mammography

MICHAEL E. HOCHMAN

> For every 2000 women invited for screening throughout 10 years, one
> will avoid dying of breast cancer and 10 healthy women, who would not
> have been diagnosed if there had not been screening, will be treated
> unnecessarily.
>
> —GØTZSCHE AND JØRGENSEN[1]

Research Question: Is screening mammography effective?[1]

Funding: The Cochrane Collaboration, an independent, nonprofit organization supported by governments, universities, hospital trusts, charities,
and donations. The Cochrane Collaboration does not accept commercial
funding.

Year Study Began: This was a meta-analysis of seven randomized trials of
screening mammography. The earliest trial began in 1963 and the most recent
began in 1991.

Year Study Published: The results of the individual trials were published during the 1970s, 1980s, 1990s, and 2000s. This review was published in 2013.

Study Location: The trials were conducted in Sweden, the United States, Canada, and the United Kingdom.

Who Was Studied: Women 39–74 years old.

How Many Patients: 599,090

Study Overview: This was a meta-analysis of randomized clinical trials of screening mammography in women without previously diagnosed breast cancer.

Which Trials Were Included: Seven high-quality trials were included in the meta-analysis. These trials are listed below with the country and start date in parentheses:

- The Health Insurance Plan trial (USA 1963)
- The Malmö trial (Sweden 1978)
- The Two-County trial (Sweden 1977)
- The Canadian trials (two trials with different age groups; Canada 1980)
- The Stockholm trial (Sweden 1981)
- The Göteborg trial (Sweden 1982)
- The United Kingdom age trial (United Kingdom 1991)

Study Intervention: In all seven trials, women were randomized to receive either an invitation for breast cancer screening with mammography or no invitation for screening. Women in the screening group were invited for two to nine rounds of screening, depending on the trial.

Follow-Up: Mean of 13 years.

Endpoints: Breast cancer mortality; all-cause mortality; surgeries (mastectomies and lumpectomies); and radiotherapy treatment.

RESULTS

- The authors judged three of the seven trials to have optimal randomization methodology; for these three trials, data were available for 292,153 women.
- Screening mammography appeared to reduce breast cancer mortality but not all-cause mortality (see Table 5.1).

- The authors calculated that approximately 30% of screen-detected breast cancers were overdiagnosed (i.e., would not have become clinically apparent or required treatment during the analysis period had it not been for screening).

Table 5.1. SUMMARY OF KEY FINDINGS

Outcome	Relative Risk with Screening (95% Confidence Intervals)
Breast Cancer Mortality	
All 7 trials	0.81 (0.74–0.87)
3 trials with optimal methodology	0.90 (0.79–1.02)
All-Cause Mortality	
All 7 trials	Unreliable[a]
3 trials with optimal methodology	0.99 (0.95–1.03)
Surgeries	
All 5 trials reporting this outcome	1.35 (1.26–1.44)
3 trials with optimal methodology	1.31 (1.22–1.44)
Radiotherapy	
All 5 trials reporting this outcome	1.32 (1.16–1.50)
1 trial with optimal methodology	1.24 (1.04–1.49)

[a] The authors felt this number was unreliable and therefore do not report it.

Criticisms and Limitations: Many of the individual trials included in this meta-analysis suffered from methodological flaws. Some of these flaws may have biased the results in favor of the screening group while others may have biased the results in favor of the controls:

- In many cases women assigned to the control groups appeared to be systematically different from those assigned to the screening groups. For example, despite efforts to exclude women with a prior diagnosis of breast cancer, in the Two-County trial it appears that some women in the control group with a prior diagnosis of breast cancer were included in the analysis. Differences such as these may have biased the results.
- Determination of breast cancer mortality rates in many of the trials was potentially biased or inaccurate. The physicians who determined the cause of death for study subjects were frequently aware of whether the subjects had been assigned to the screening versus control groups, and it is possible that their judgments were influenced by this knowledge. Furthermore, few autopsies of patients who died were

performed, and therefore many of the cause-of-death determinations
may have been inaccurate.

- Some experts have criticized the screening mammography
  trials because, particularly in some of the trials, women in the
  control groups began receiving screening before the trials were
  concluded. Because it presumably takes several years before the
  benefits of screening are apparent, it is unlikely this would have
  substantially affected the trial results. Still, it is possible that
  mammograms among controls partially obscured the benefits of
  screening.
- Some women in these trials received one-view mammograms rather
  than the standard two-view studies. It is possible that the one-view
  films were less effective at identifying cancers.
- These trials were all conducted several years ago. Breast cancer
  treatments have improved in recent years, and some experts believe
  that with current treatment options, the benefits of early detection of
  breast cancer may be smaller.[2]

Other Relevant Studies and Information:

- A modeling study suggests that screening mammography every
  2 years "achieves most of the benefit of annual screening with less
  harm." In addition, this study suggests that screening mammograms
  in women between the ages of 40 to 49 lead to only a small benefit but
  a high rate of false positive results.[3]
- A 25-year follow-up analysis of the Canadian trial, which involved
  almost 90,000 women, concluded that "annual mammography in
  women aged 40–59 does not reduce mortality from breast cancer
  beyond that of physical examination or usual care when adjuvant
  therapy for breast cancer is freely available." The analysis also
  suggested that 22% of "screen detected invasive breast cancers were
  over-diagnosed, representing one over-diagnosed breast cancer for
  every 424 women" receiving screening.[4]
- Based on the results of this analysis and others, in 2014 the Swiss
  Medical Board recommended against continuing the country's
  mammography screening program.[5]
- Table 5.2 lists breast cancer screening guidelines from two major
  organizations.

Table 5.2. MAJOR BREAST CANCER SCREENING GUIDELINES

Guideline	Recommendations
The US Preventive Services Task Force	• Screening recommended every 2 years for women 50–74 years of age • "The decision to start [screening] before the age of 50 years should be an individual one and take patient context into account . . ."
The American Cancer Society	• Yearly mammograms are recommended starting at age 40 and continuing for as long as a woman is in good health

Summary and Implications: Most of the trials of screening mammography have considerable methodological flaws. Despite these limitations, the Cochrane Review suggests that screening mammography modestly reduces breast cancer mortality but may not reduce all-cause mortality. In addition, screening mammography leads to the diagnosis and unnecessary treatment of a substantial number of women who may never have developed symptoms of breast cancer. According to the authors, for every 2,000 women offered screening mammograms over a 10-year period, one will avoid dying from breast cancer while 10 will be treated for breast cancer unnecessarily. The appropriate use of screening mammography remains an area of considerable controversy.

CLINICAL CASE: SCREENING MAMMOGRAPHY

Case History:
A 68-year-old woman with chronic obstructive pulmonary disease, diabetes, and osteoporosis visits your clinic for a routine visit. When you mention that she is due for a screening mammogram, she protests: "I have so many other medical problems. Why do we need to look for more?"

Based on the results of the Cochrane Review on mammography, what can you tell this patient about the risks and benefits of screening mammography?

Suggested Answer:
The Cochrane Mammography review suggests that screening mammography modestly reduces breast cancer mortality but may not reduce all-cause mortality. In addition, screening mammography leads to the diagnosis and unnecessary treatment of a substantial number of women who may never have developed symptoms of breast cancer. Some women may not feel that this trade-off is worth it.

The woman in this vignette has other significant comorbidities and does not want to "look for more." Thus, it would be perfectly reasonable for her to opt not to undergo screening. Since this patient is in poor health, screening may not even be appropriate for her since the benefits of screening occur several years down the road and she may not live long enough to realize these benefits. Indeed, the American Cancer Society only recommends screening among women in good overall health.

References

1. Gøtzsche PC, Jørgensen KJ. Screening for breast cancer with mammography. *Cochrane Database Syst Rev.* 2013 Jun 4;6:CD001877.
2. Welch HG. Screening mammography—a long run for a short slide? *N Engl J Med.* 2010;363(13):1276–1278.
3. Mandelblatt JS et al. Effects of mammography screening under different screening schedules: model estimates of potential benefits and harms. *Ann Intern Med.* 2009;151:738–747.
4. Miller AB et al. Twenty-five-year follow-up for breast cancer incidence and mortality of the Canadian National Breast Screening Study: randomised screening trial. *BMJ.* 2014 Feb 11;348:g366.
5. Biller-Andorno N, Jüni P. Abolishing mammography screening programs? A view from the Swiss Medical Board. *N Engl J Med.* 2014 May 22;370(21):1965–1967.

6

The European Randomized Study of Screening for Prostate Cancer (ERSPC)

MICHAEL E. HOCHMAN

[The ERSPC showed] a relative reduction of 21% in the rate of death from prostate cancer in the screening group . . . [but this] reduction was achieved after considerable use of resources . . . [and there was no] significant between-group difference in all-cause mortality.

—DR. ANTHONY B. MILLER[1]

Research Question: Is screening for prostate cancer with prostate-specific-antigen (PSA) testing effective?[2,3]

Funding: Europe Against Cancer, the European Union, local grants, and an unrestricted grant from Beckman Coulter, which manufactures PSA tests.

Year Study Began: 1991

Year Study Published: 2012

Study Location: Numerous sites in seven European countries (The Netherlands, Belgium, Sweden, Finland, Italy, Spain, and Switzerland)

Who Was Studied: Men between the ages of 55 and 69.

How Many Patients: 162,388

Study Overview: See Figure 6.1 for a summary of the study's design.

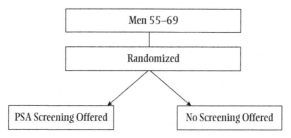

Figure 6.1 Summary of the Study Design.

Study Intervention: The study protocols varied slightly from country to country. In the screening group, men were typically offered screening every 4 years, and most were only screened with a PSA test (though some men also received a digital rectal examination and/or transrectal ultrasound). Men with a PSA ≥3.0 ng/mL were typically referred for prostate biopsy; however, in some countries a higher cutoff (typically 4.0 ng/mL) was used. Most men who underwent biopsies received sextant (six-core) biopsies guided by transrectal ultrasonography. Men with positive biopsies were treated at the discretion of their physicians, that is, no standard treatment protocols were specified.

In the control group, men were not invited for PSA screening as part of the trial, though a small percentage may have received PSA screening outside of the study protocol.

Follow-Up: Median of 11 years.

Endpoints: Primary outcome: Death from prostate cancer. Secondary outcomes: Prostate cancer diagnoses, all-cause mortality.

RESULTS

- 82.2% of men in the screening group were screened at least once (i.e., 17.8% declined screening), and those who were screened received an average of 2.3 screenings.
- 16.6% of screening tests were positive (i.e., PSA ≥3.0).
- 85.9% of men who had a positive screening test agreed to undergo biopsy, and 24.1% of men who underwent a biopsy were found to have cancer.

- In total, 9.6% of men in the screening group were diagnosed with prostate cancer versus 6.0% of men in the control group.
- Prostate cancers detected in the screening group were less advanced (lower stage and Gleason score) than those detected in the control group.
- The authors calculated that 936 men would need to be offered screening and 33 additional men would need to be diagnosed with prostate cancer to prevent one death from prostate cancer (including all available follow-up data for ≥12 years).
- There was a reduction in prostate cancer mortality in the screening group relative to the control group but no difference in all-cause mortality between the groups (see Table 6.1).

Table 6.1. SUMMARY OF KEY FINDINGS[a]

Outcome	Screening Group	Control Group	P Value
Prostate Cancer Mortality	0.39	0.50	0.001
All-Cause Mortality	18.2	18.5	0.50

[a] Event rates are per 1,000 person-years, that is, the number of deaths that occurred for every 1,000 years of participant time. For example, 0.39 deaths per 1,000 person-years means that, on average, there were 0.39 deaths among 100 subjects who were each enrolled in the trial for 10 years.

Criticisms and Limitations: It is likely that some men (approximately 20%) in the control group received prostate cancer screening from their physicians outside of the study protocol (referred to as "contamination"). The authors did not estimate the rate at which contamination occurred; however, if it occurred frequently it would have led to an underestimation of both the benefits and harms of screening.

This was a preliminary report from the ERSPC trial, which is ongoing. Future analyses will provide long-term follow-up data. It is possible that the impact of screening may be more favorable with longer follow-up. Indeed, recently reported results after 13 years of follow up suggest a slightly more favorable benefit vs. risk profile of screening (see below).

Men in this study were generally screened every 4 years; however, in many countries (including historically in the United States) men are screened more frequently (e.g., every 1 to 2 years). More frequent screening would presumably improve the benefits of screening but would also increase harms from false positive results (i.e., overdiagnosis and overtreatment of early-stage cancers that would never cause harm in the patient's lifetime).

Most men with positive screening tests in the study underwent sextant (six-core) biopsies. However, many urologists now recommend extended core biopsies in which a larger portion of the prostate is sampled. While extended

core biopsies increase the sensitivity for prostate cancer, they are also associated with more false positive results.

The study was not adequately powered to detect small reductions in all-cause
mortality between the screening and control groups.

Other Relevant Studies and Information:

- Early stage prostate cancer is commonly treated with surgery or radiation
  therapy (though a strategy of close monitoring with "active surveillance"
  is also a recommended approach). Complications of surgery and radiation
  include urinary incontinence, sexual dysfunction, and bowel problems.
- A simulation analysis using data from the ERSPC trial suggested that
  overdiagnosis and overtreatment of prostate cancer as a result of screening
  may adversely impact quality of life, at least partially counterbalancing the
  benefits of prostate cancer screening.[4]
- A 13 year follow-up analysis of the ERSPC data suggest that with longer
  follow-up screening the overall impact of screening becomes slightly more
  favorable. After 13 years, the rate of prostate cancer death was 0.43 per 1,000
  person years in the screening group vs. 0.54 among controls. The authors of
  this analysis calculated that 781 men would need to be offered screening and 27
  additional men would need to be diagnosed with prostate cancer to prevent one
  death from prostate cancer. Again, there was no all-cause mortality benefit.[5]
- Fourteen-year follow-up data were reported from one of the sites where this
  trial took place. Data from this site, where patients were screened every 2 years,
  showed a more substantial reduction in prostate cancer deaths (just 293 men
  needed to be screened and 12 diagnosed with prostate cancer to prevent one
  prostate cancer death). There was no reduction in all-cause mortality, however.[6]
- Another large randomized trial in the United States did not show a benefit
  of prostate cancer screening with annual PSA measurements and digital
  rectal examination. However, some patients in the control group received
  screening from their physicians outside of the study protocol, which may
  have affected the results.[7,8]
- In 2012, the US Preventive Services Task Force developed new guidelines
  recommending against routine prostate cancer screening because the potential
  harms from screening (unnecessary surgeries and radiation therapy) may not
  outweigh the small benefits.[9] A guidance statement from the American College of
  Physicians indicates that clinicians should discuss the "limited potential benefits
  and substantial harms of screening for prostate cancer" with men 50–69 years old
  and that "clinicians should not screen for prostate cancer using the prostate-specific
  antigen test in patients who do not express a clear preference for screening."[10]

Summary and Implications: Screening for prostate cancer with PSA testing
every 4 years leads to a small but significant reduction in prostate cancer deaths
along with a substantial increase in the (potentially unnecessary) diagnosis

and treatment of prostate cancer. There was no effect of screening on all-cause mortality, though the study was not powered for this analysis. The ERSPC trial is ongoing, and future analyses will provide longer term follow-up data. In the meantime, guidelines from the US Preventive Services Task Force recommend against routine screening.

CLINICAL CASE: SCREENING FOR PROSTATE CANCER

Case History:
A 50-year-old African American man whose father died from prostate cancer at the age of 64 presents to your clinic for a routine evaluation. Based on the results of the ERSPC trial, do you recommend prostate cancer screening for this patient?

Suggested Answer:
The ERSPC trial found that screening for prostate cancer with PSA testing every 4 years leads to a small reduction in prostate cancer deaths along with a substantial increase in the (potentially unnecessary) diagnosis and treatment of prostate cancer. There was no effect of screening on all-cause mortality, though the study was not powered for this analysis. Based on the results of ERSPC and a large US prostate cancer screening trial, guidelines from the US Preventive Services Task Force recommend against routine screening.

However, the patient in this vignette is at particularly high risk for developing prostate cancer (African American men, as well as men with a family history of prostate cancer, are at increased risk). For this reason, some experts might advocate screening for this patient.

On the other hand, there is no evidence to suggest that PSA screening is any more effective for identifying dangerous cancers among high-risk patients. In fact, since PSA levels tend to be higher among African American men than among white men, it is possible that the man in this vignette would be at particularly high risk for being inappropriately diagnosed with a slow-growing prostate cancer that would never impact his life. (The percentage of patients in ERSPC who were African American or who had a family history of prostate cancer was not specified.)

Thus, there is no correct answer to the question of whether or not this patient should be screened. You might inform this man that prostate cancer screening is no longer recommended for most men. However, it would be reasonable to consider screening in his case because he is at increased risk. Should he express an interest in screening, you should inform him of the associated risks (the potentially unnecessary diagnosis and treatment of a slow-growing cancer that otherwise would not impact his life) before proceeding.

References

1. Miller AB. New data on prostate-cancer mortality after PSA screening. *N Engl J Med*. 2012;366(11):1047–1048.

2. Schröder FH et al. Screening and prostate-cancer mortality in a randomized European study. *N Engl J Med*. 2009;360(13):1320–1328.

3. Schröder FH et al. Prostate-cancer mortality at 11 years of follow-up. *N Engl J Med*. 2012;366(11):981–990.

4. Heijnsdijk EA et al. Quality-of-life effects of prostate-specific antigen screening. *N Engl J Med*. 2012;367(7):595–605.

5. Schröder FH, Hugosson J, Roobol MJ, Tammela TL, Zappa M, Nelen V, Kwiatkowski M, Lujan M, Määttänen L, Lilja H, Denis LJ, Recker F, Paez A, Bangma CH, Carlsson S, Puliti D, Villers A, Rebillard X, Hakama M, Stenman UH, Kujala P, Taari K, Aus G, Huber A, van der Kwast TH, van Schaik RH, de Koning HJ, Moss SM, Auvinen A; for the ERSPC Investigators. Screening and prostate cancer mortality: results of the European Randomised Study of Screening for Prostate Cancer (ERSPC) at 13 years of follow-up. *Lancet*. 2014 Aug 6. pii: S0140-6736(14)60525-0.

6. Hugosson J et al. Mortality results from the Göteborg randomised population-based prostate-cancer screening trial. *Lancet Oncol*. 2010;11(8):725–732.

7. Andriole GL et al. Mortality results from a randomized prostate-cancer screening trial. *N Engl J Med*. 2009;360:1310–1319.

8. Andriole GL et al. Prostate cancer screening in the randomized Prostate, Lung, Colorectal, and Ovarian Cancer Screening Trial: mortality results after 13 years of follow-up. *J Natl Cancer Inst*. 2012;104:1–8.

9. Chou R et al. Screening for Prostate Cancer: A Review of the Evidence for the U.S. Preventive Services Task Force. *Ann Intern Med*. 2011;155(11):762–771.

10. Qaseem A et al. Clinical Guidelines Committee of the American College of Physicians. Screening for prostate cancer: a guidance statement from the Clinical Guidelines Committee of the American College of Physicians. *Ann Intern Med*. 2013;158(10):761.

7

Screening for Lung Cancer with Low-Dose Computed Tomography versus Chest Radiography

The National Lung Screening Trial (NLST)

KATHRYN WHITE

In the [National Lung Cancer Screening Trial], a 20.0% [relative] decrease in mortality from lung cancer was observed in the low-dose CT group ... [however] the reduction in lung-cancer mortality must be weighed against the harms from [false] positive screening results and overdiagnosis, as well as the costs.

— NATIONAL LUNG SCREENING TRIAL INVESTIGATORS[1]

Research Question: In older individuals with an extensive smoking history, does screening with low-dose computed tomography (CT) reduce mortality from lung cancer compared to single-view chest radiography?[1]

Funding: National Cancer Institute.

Year Study Began: 2002

Year Study Published: 2011

Study Location: 33 medical centers in the United States.

Who Was Studied: Current or former smokers 55 to 74 years of age with a minimum 30 pack-year cigarette smoking history. Former smokers were required to have quit smoking within 15 years of randomization.

Who Was Excluded: Those with a history of lung cancer or clinical suspicion of lung cancer (e.g., hemoptysis or unintentional weight loss), and those with a chest CT within 18 months of enrollment were excluded.

How Many Patients: 53,454

Study Overview: See Figure 7.1 for a summary of the study's design.

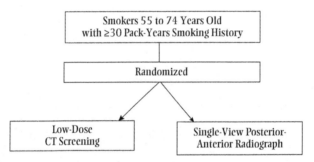

Figure 7.1 Summary of the Study Design.

Study Intervention: Participants received screening with either low-dose CT or chest radiography at the time of enrollment and then yearly for 2 years (total of three annual screenings per participant). Participants were discouraged from undergoing screening procedures outside of the study. All CT scans were performed on multidetector scanners and had an average effective radiation dose of 1.5 mSv (diagnostic CT scans have an average effective dose of 8 mSv).

Positive screens on low-dose CT included those demonstrating noncalcified nodules ≥4 mm and on chest radiographs as showing any noncalcified nodule or mass. Adenopathy, pleural effusion, or other findings suggestive of lung cancer could be defined as a positive screen at the discretion of the interpreting radiologist.

Screening results were sent to the participant and his or her provider within 4 weeks. Guidelines for the workup of positive screenings were developed trial-wide, but not mandated by the protocol.

Follow-Up: Median of 6.5 years.

Endpoints: Primary outcome: Lung cancer mortality. Secondary outcomes: All-cause mortality rate and rate of lung cancer diagnosis.

RESULTS

- Adherence to screening was high in both groups (95% in the low-dose CT group and 93% in the chest radiography group).
- During all three rounds of screening, there was a substantially higher rate of positive screens in the low-dose CT group compared to the chest radiography group (Table 7.1). Positivity rates noticeably decreased at the second screen in both groups.
- Diagnostic workups typically involved additional imaging and occasionally invasive diagnostic procedures; complication rates from diagnostic workups were similar between groups (1.4% in the low-dose CT group versus 1.6% in the chest radiograph group).
- Rates of lung cancer in the low-dose CT group were higher when compared to the chest radiography group (Table 7.2).
- Across all rounds, diagnostic workups revealed cancer in 3.6% of positive screens in the low-dose CT group and 5.5% of positive screens in the chest radiography group.
- There were fewer interval cancers (cancers diagnosed outside of the screening protocol), in the low-dose CT group (N = 44) than in the chest radiography group (N = 137).
- In the low-dose CT group, there were more total stage IA lung cancers and fewer total stage IV cancers than in the chest radiography group, reflecting a shift toward the diagnosis of earlier stage cancers with CT screening.
- Lung cancer mortality was lower in the low-dose CT group compared to the chest radiography group (Table 7.2).
- All-cause mortality was reduced by 6.7% in the low-dose CT group compared to the chest radiography group ($P = 0.02$) with 60.3% of the excess deaths in the chest radiography group caused by lung cancer.

Table 7.1. RATES OF POSITIVE SCREENING TESTS IN TRIAL

	Percentage of Subjects with at Least One Positive Screen
Low-Dose CT Group	39.1
Chest Radiography Group	16.0

Table 7.2. SUMMARY OF KEY FINDINGS

	Low-Dose CT Group	Chest Radiography Group	Comparison Measure
Lung Cancer Diagnosis	645 cases per 100,000 person-years	572 cases per 100,000 person-years	Odds ratio of 1.13 (1.03, 1.23)
Lung Cancer Mortality	247 deaths per 100,000 person-years	309 deaths per 100,000 person-years	Relative risk reduction of 20.0% (6.8, 26.7)

Criticisms and Limitations: Improvements in contemporary CT scanners may yield better diagnostic resolution at lower radiation doses compared to those used in the NLST. The results in this trial may not be reproducible in the general community since the NLST centers had expertise in radiology and the treatment of lung cancer. Implementation on the national level will require standardization of methods, similar expertise, and a multidisciplinary approach to ensure optimal benefits to risks. Finally, there was no control group that received no screening; however, other large trials comparing chest radiography with no screening have found no benefits of screening with chest radiography.

Other Relevant Studies and Information:

- In a follow-up analysis of the NLST data it was estimated that almost 20% of cancers diagnosed by CT screening would not have become clinically apparent after 6.4 years of follow-up.[2] The proportion of such cancers may decrease with longer follow-up or if different criteria are used to identify positive screens, however.
- A subset of 2,812 patients from the NLST completed questionnaires assessing health-related quality of life and anxiety levels before and after screening. While patients with true positive screening results demonstrated reduced health-related quality of life and increased anxiety levels compared to other participants, there was no difference observed between patients with false positive or significant incidental findings and those with negative screens.[3]
- Smaller European trials have compared low-dose CT scans to a control group of usual care (as opposed to chest radiography as in the NLST) and have also demonstrated a modest benefit from screening.[4,5,6]

- The US Preventive Services Task Force provides a Grade B rating for yearly lung cancer screening with low-dose CT in persons 55–80 years old and a smoking history of ≥30 pack-years. Screening should be discontinued once the patient has not smoked for 15 years or with the development of a health problem that substantially limits life expectancy.[7]

Summary and Implications: The NLST demonstrated a 20% relative reduction in lung cancer mortality and a small but significant overall mortality benefit from lung cancer screening with low-dose CT among a group of high-risk smokers. Using the NLST criteria, roughly 320 such patients would need to be screened to prevent one death from lung cancer. Based on the results of the NLST, new guidelines from the US Preventive Services Task Force recommend yearly lung cancer screening with low-dose CT in persons at high risk for lung cancer based on age and smoking history.

CLINICAL CASE: LOW-DOSE CT SCREENING

Case History:
A 63-year-old man with chronic obstructive lung disease and hypertension presents for a routine visit. He has smoked one pack of cigarettes per day from the ages of 16 to 55. Based on the results of the NLST, would you recommend that this patient undergo screening for lung cancer with a low-dose CT?

Suggested Answer:
The NLST demonstrated a reduction in lung cancer deaths with yearly low-dose CTs in patients at high risk for lung cancer based on smoking history. Based on this patient's 39 pack-year smoking history and recent quit date, he fits the inclusion criteria of this study and should be considered for yearly lung cancer screening with a low-dose CT. The clinician should discuss with the patient the benefits of screening, including the possibility of reducing mortality from lung cancer, but also the potential harms of high false positivity rates such as complications of follow-up testing and the potential to overtreat indolent cancers that may never become relevant during that patient's lifetime. Finally, the critical importance of smoking cessation and durable abstinence must be stressed at every patient visit and in conjunction with screening.

Based on an understanding of the risks and benefits of screening, the patient should ultimately decide whether or not to undergo screening. If he opts for screening, recommendations from the US Preventive Services Task Force suggest yearly screening until the patient has not been smoking for 15 years or develops a health problem that substantially limits life expectancy or the ability or willingness to undergo potentially curative lung surgery.

References

1. National Lung Screening Trial Research Team. Reduced lung-cancer mortality with low-dose computed tomographic screening. *N Engl J Med.* 2011;365(5):395–409.
2. Patz EF Jr et al. Overdiagnosis in low-dose computed tomography screening for lung cancer. *JAMA Intern Med.* 2014;174:269–274.
3. Gareen IF et al. Short-term impact of lung cancer screening on participant health-related quality of life and state anxiety in the National Lung Screening Trial. *Cancer.* 2014. In press.
4. Infante M et al. A randomized study of lung cancer screening with spiral computed tomography: three-year results from DANTE trial. *Am J Respir Crit Care Med.* 2009;180(5):445–453.
5. Saghir Z et al. CT screening for lung cancer brings forward early disease. The randomized Danish Lung Cancer Screening Trial: status after five annual screening rounds with low-dose CT. *Thorax.* 2012;67(4):296–301.
6. Pastorino U et al. Annual or biannual CT screening versus observation in heavy smokers: 5-year results of the MILD trial. *Eur J Cancer Prev.* 2012;21(3):308–315.
7. US Preventive Services Task Force. Recommendation statement: screening for lung cancer. http://www.uspreventiveservicestaskforce.org/uspstf13/lungcan/lungcanfinalrs.htm. Accessed on February 8, 2014. *Ann Intern Med.* Published online 2013 Dec 31; doi:10.7326/M13-2771

Endocrinology

8

Treating Elevated Blood Sugar Levels in Patients with Type 2 Diabetes

The United Kingdom Prospective Diabetes Study (UKPDS)

MICHAEL E. HOCHMAN

> UKPDS shows that an intensive glucose-control treatment policy that maintains . . . [a hemoglobin A1c of 7.0%–7.4%] substantially reduces the frequency of [diabetes-related complications].
>
> —THE UKPDS STUDY GROUP[1]

Research Question: Does treating type 2 diabetes with medications to lower the blood sugar reduce diabetes-related complications more than dietary therapy alone?[1,2]

Funding: The United Kingdom Medical Research Council and other public funding agencies from the United Kingdom; the US National Institutes of Health; several charitable organizations; and several pharmaceutical companies.

Year Study Began: 1977

Year Study Published: 1998

Study Location: Patients were referred from numerous general practitioner clinics in the United Kingdom.

Who Was Studied: Patients 25–65 with newly diagnosed type 2 diabetes. Patients were required to have a fasting plasma glucose >108 mg/dL on two mornings, 1 to 3 weeks apart.

Who Was Excluded: Patients with a serum creatinine >2.0 mg/dL, those with a myocardial infarction within the previous year, those with angina or heart failure, those with retinopathy requiring laser treatment, and those with a concurrent illness limiting life expectancy.

How Many Patients: 4,209

Study Overview: A group of 2,505 patients (both overweight and nonoverweight) were randomized to receive either intensive treatment with insulin or a sulfonylurea, or to dietary therapy alone. A group of 1,704 overweight patients were randomized to receive either intensive treatment with metformin, intensive treatment with insulin or a sulfonylurea, or dietary therapy alone. Figure 8.1 summarizes the treatment allocation.

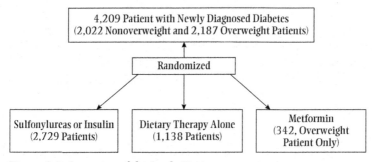

Figure 8.1 Summary of the Study Design.

Study Intervention: Patients in the dietary therapy group received counseling from a dietician. Patients in the sulfonylureas/insulin group and in the metformin group received both counseling and medications.

All medications were titrated for a target fasting blood glucose of <108 mg/ dL. Patients in the insulin group were initially started on basal insulin, and prandial insulin was added if the daily dose was >14 units or if the premeal or bedtime glucose was >126 mg/dL. Patients in the sulfonylureas group received chlorpropamide, glibenclamide, or glipizide. Patients in the metformin group were started on metformin 850 mg once daily, which could be increased to a maximum of 1,700 mg in the morning and 850 mg at night.

Patients in the dietary, sulfonylureas, and metformin groups who developed symptoms of hyperglycemia (thirst or polyuria) or who had glucose levels >270 mg/dL were started on additional medications.

Follow-Up: A median of 10.0 years in the sulfonylureas/insulin group and 10.7 years in the metformin group.

Endpoints:

1. Diabetes-related endpoints: Sudden death, death from hyperglycemia or hypoglycemia, myocardial infarction, angina, heart failure, stroke, renal failure, amputation, and ophthalmologic complications
2. Diabetes-related deaths: Sudden death or death due to myocardial infarction, peripheral vascular disease, renal disease, hyperglycemia, or hypoglycemia
3. All-cause mortality
4. Microvascular disease: Vitreous hemorrhage, retinal photocoagulation, or renal failure

RESULTS

Sulfonylureas/Insulin versus Dietary Therapy

- After treatment, the median hemoglobin A1c (HbA1c) was 7.0% in the sulfonylureas/insulin group versus 7.9% in the dietary group.
- There were more hypoglycemic episodes in the sulfonylureas/insulin group than in the dietary group.
- Patients in the sulfonylureas/insulin group gained an average of 2.9 kg more weight than those in the dietary group.
- Patients in the sulfonylureas and insulin group experienced fewer diabetes-related complications and less microvascular disease than patients in the dietary group (see Table 8.1).

Table 8.1. SUMMARY OF KEY FINDINGS[a]

Outcome	Sulfonylureas and Insulin Group (N = 2,729)	Dietary Group (N = 1,138)	P Value
Diabetes-Related Endpoints	40.9	46.0	0.03
Diabetes-Related Deaths	10.4	11.5	0.34
All-Cause Mortality	17.9	18.9	0.44
Microvascular Disease	8.6	11.4	0.01

[a] Event rates are per 1,000 person-years, that is, the number of events that occurred for every 1,000 years of participant time. For example, 40.9 events per 1,000 person-years means that there were, on average, 40.9 events among 100 subjects who were each enrolled in the trial for 10 years.

Metformin versus Dietary Therapy and Sulfonylureas/Insulin (Overweight Patients)

- After treatment, the median HbA1c was 7.4% in the metformin group versus 8.0% in the dietary group (patients in the sulfonylureas/insulin group had similar HbA1c levels, as those in the metformin group, though the actual level was not reported).
- There were more hypoglycemic episodes among patients in the metformin group than among patients in the dietary therapy group. However, patients in the insulin/sulfonylureas group had the highest rate of hypoglycemic episodes.
- Patients in the metformin and dietary therapy groups had similar changes in body weight, while patients in the sulfonylureas/insulin group gained more weight than those in the metformin and dietary therapy groups.
- Obese patients in the metformin group had fewer diabetes-related complications than patients in both the dietary group and the sulfonylureas and insulin group (see Table 8.2).

Table 8.2. KEY FINDINGS AMONG OVERWEIGHT PATIENTS[a]

Outcome	Metformin Group (N = 342)	Dietary Group (N = 411)	Sulfonylureas and Insulin Group (N = 951)	P Value[b]
Diabetes-Related Endpoints	29.8	43.8	40.1	0.0023, 0.0034
Diabetes-Related Deaths	7.5	12.7	10.3	0.017, nonsignificant[c]
All-Cause Mortality	13.5	20.6	18.9	0.011, 0.021
Microvascular Disease	6.7	9.2	7.7	0.19, nonsignificant[c]

[a] Event rates are per 1,000 person-years.
[b] Metformin versus dietary; metformin versus sulfonylureas/insulin.
[c] Actual P values not reported.

Criticisms and Limitations: UKPDS did not define appropriate HbA1c targets for patients with type 2 diabetes.

Other Relevant Studies and Information:
At the completion of the UKPDS trial, patients were managed for diabetes by their physicians. However, they continued to be monitored by the UKPDS researchers for an additional 10 years. After a median of 16.8 years of follow-up in the sulfonylureas/insulin group and 17.7 years of follow-up in the metformin group, long-term outcomes were reported:[3]

- Within a year of the trial's completion, average HbA1c levels were similar among all groups.
- Patients in the sulfonylureas/insulin group still had fewer diabetes-related endpoints and less microvascular disease than those in the dietary group.
- Patients in the sulfonylureas/insulin group had fewer myocardial infarctions and lower diabetes-related and all-cause mortality than those in the dietary group, findings that were not present in the initial analysis.
- Overweight patients in the metformin group still had fewer diabetes-related endpoints, diabetes-related mortality, and all-cause mortality than those in the dietary group.

The UKPDS trial also compared tight blood pressure control with an ACE inhibitor and beta blocker (target blood pressure <150/85 mm Hg) versus more lenient control (target blood pressure <180/105 mm Hg) among patients in the trial who had hypertension. Patients in the tight blood pressure control group had a reduction in total diabetes-related endpoints, diabetes-related death, stroke, and microvascular disease.[4] A follow-up analysis 10 years after the trial stopped did not demonstrate sustained benefits, however, suggesting that "good blood-pressure control must be continued if the benefits are to be maintained."[5]

Other important studies examining glycemic control among patients with type 2 diabetes are described in the summary of the ACCORD trial (see Chapter 9). The benefits of tight blood sugar control in type 1 diabetes are explored in the summary of the DCCT trial (see Chapter 10).

Summary and Implications: The UKPDS trial was the first study to conclusively show the benefits of medications for treating elevated blood sugar in patients with type 2 diabetes. Patients receiving sulfonylureas, insulin, and metformin had fewer diabetes-related complications than patients assigned to dietary therapy alone. The benefits of medications persisted 10 years after the trial was stopped.

CLINICAL CASE: TREATING ELEVATED BLOOD SUGAR LEVELS IN PATIENTS WITH TYPE 2 DIABETES

Case History:
A 36-year-old woman presents to your clinic with newly diagnosed type 2 diabetes. She is overweight with a body mass index of 36 kg/m^2 and does not exercise. Her HbA1c is 7.8%. Based on the results of the UKPDS trial, do you want to start this patient on medications to treat her elevated blood sugar?

Suggested Answer:
The UKPDS trial was the first study to conclusively show the benefits of medications for treating elevated blood sugar in patients with type 2 diabetes. Patients receiving sulfonylureas, insulin, and metformin had fewer diabetes-related complications than patients assigned to dietary therapy alone.

The patient in this vignette is very young, however, and her HbA1c is only mildly elevated. While it would not be unreasonable to start her on a medication—probably metformin—an argument could also be made to encourage her to implement lifestyle changes first. If she were able to lose a considerable amount of weight and begin exercising, it is likely that her diabetes would improve and she might no longer require medications.

References

1. UK Prospective Diabetes Study Group. Intensive blood-glucose control with sulphonylureas or insulin compared with conventional treatment and risk of complications in patients with type 2 diabetes (UKPDS 33). *Lancet.* 1998;352(9131):837–853.
2. UK Prospective Diabetes Study Group. Effect of intensive blood-glucose control with metformin on complications in overweight patients with type 2 diabetes (UKPDS 34). *Lancet.* 1998;352(9131):854–865.
3. Holman RR et al. Ten-year follow-up of intensive glucose control in type 2 diabetes. *N Engl J Med.* 2008;359:2049–2056.
4. UK Prospective Diabetes Study Group. Tight blood pressure control and risk of macrovascular and microvascular complications in type 2 diabetes: UKPDS 38. UK Prospective Diabetes Study Group. *BMJ.* 1998;317(7160):703–713.
5. Holman RR et al. Long-term follow-up after tight control of blood pressure in type 2 diabetes. *N Engl J Med.* 2008;359(15):1565–1576.

Intensive versus Conservative Blood Sugar Control in Patients with Type 2 Diabetes

The ACCORD Trial

MICHAEL E. HOCHMAN

> One message that has been pushed down our throats for over twenty years at least is that the lower your blood glucose levels are the better... The surprising results of the [ACCORD trial are] that . . . there were more deaths in the intensive therapy group than in the standard therapy group.
>
> —DR. DAVID MCCULLOCH
> *Clinical Professor of Medicine*
> *University of Washington*

Research Question: Should doctors target a "normal" blood glucose level in patients with type 2 diabetes?[1]

Funding: The National Heart, Lung, and Blood Institute (NHLBI).

Year Study Began: 2001

Year Study Published: 2008

Study Location: 77 centers in the United States and Canada.

Who Was Studied: Patients 40–79 years old with type 2 diabetes, a hemoglobin A1c (HbA1c) ≥7.5%, and known cardiovascular disease or risk factors.

Who Was Excluded: Patients who were unwilling to do home blood glucose monitoring or unwilling to inject insulin; patients with frequent hypoglycemic episodes; and patients with a creatinine >1.5 mg/dL.

How Many Patients: 10,251

Study Overview: See Figure 9.1 for a summary of the ACCORD study's design.

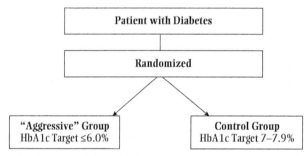

Figure 9.1 Summary of the Study Design.

Study Intervention: Physicians could use any available diabetes medications to achieve the blood glucose targets. Metformin was used in 60% of the patients, insulin in 35%, and sulfonylureas in 50%.

Follow-Up: Mean of 3.5 years.

Endpoints: Primary outcome: A composite of nonfatal myocardial infarction, nonfatal stroke, or death from cardiovascular causes. Secondary outcome: All-cause mortality.

RESULTS

- The mean baseline HbA1c in both groups was 8.1%.
- The mean post-treatment HbA1c in the "aggressive" group was 6.4% versus 7.5% in the control group.
- The mean weight gain in the "aggressive" group was 3.5 kg versus 0.4 kg in the control group.
- See Table 9.1 for a summary of the ACCORD study's findings.

Table 9.1. SUMMARY OF KEY FINDINGS

Outcome	"Aggressive" Group	Control Group	P Value
Hypoglycemia Requiring Medical Assistance	10.5%	3.5%	<0.001
Cardiovascular Events or Cardiac Death	6.9%	7.2%	0.16
All-Cause Mortality	5.0%	4.0%	0.04

Criticisms and Limitations: The study only included patients with cardiovascular disease or risk factors, and it does not provide information about which medications may have been responsible for the excess mortality in the "aggressive group."

Other Relevant Studies and Information:

- The increased mortality rate among patients in the "aggressive" group persisted after 5 years of follow-up.[2]
- Another report involving the ACCORD data showed that, despite the increased mortality, patients in the "aggressive" group had lower rates of early-stage microvascular disease ("albuminuria and some eye complications and neuropathy").[3]
- The Veteran's Affairs Diabetes Trial (VADT) compared "aggressive" blood glucose management (targeting "normal" blood glucose levels) with standard glucose management and found no benefit of the aggressive approach.[4]
- The ADVANCE trial found that patients treated for an HbA1c target of 6.5% had lower rates of diabetes-related complications, primarily nephropathy, than did patients treated for a standard HbA1c target.[5]
- Most clinical practice guidelines recommend an HbA1c targets of <6.5%–7.0%, and less aggressive targets for patients at high risk for hypoglycemia such as the elderly.[6,7]

Summary and Implications: In ACCORD, a target HbA1c of ≤6.0% was associated with increased mortality compared with a target of 7.0%–7.9%. Targeting an HbA1c ≤6.0% was associated with reduced early-stage microvascular disease, however. The optimal HbA1c target in patients with diabetes remains an area of active investigation.

CLINICAL CASE: INTENSIVE VERSUS CONSERVATIVE BLOOD SUGAR CONTROL

Case History:

A 60-year-old woman with long-standing type 2 diabetes, hypertension, and hyperlipidemia presents for a routine office visit. Her diabetes medications include metformin 1,000 mg twice daily, insulin glargine 40 units at bedtime, and regular insulin 12 units prior to each meal. She proudly shows you her blood sugar log, which demonstrates excellent sugar control, with fasting morning sugars averaging 82. Her most recent HbA1c is 6.4%. Her only concerns are her continued inability to lose weight and occasional episodes of "shaking" when her blood sugars drop below 75.

After reading the ACCORD trial, what adjustments might you make to her diabetes medications?

Suggested Answer:

The ACCORD trial showed that aggressive blood sugar management with a target HbA1c of ≤6.0% was associated with increased mortality. In addition, targeting an HbA1c of ≤6.0% led to weight gain and an increased rate of hypoglycemic episodes. This patient's HbA1c is 6.4%—which was the mean HbA1c level in patients assigned to the "aggressive" blood sugar group in ACCORD. Thus, this patient's blood sugar control is probably too tight, and her insulin dose (either the insulin glargine, regular insulin, or both depending on her blood sugar patterns) should be reduced. This change would be expected to reduce the frequency of her hypoglycemic episodes, make it easier for her to lose weight, and perhaps reduce her risk of death.

References

1. Action to Control Cardiovascular Risk in Diabetes Study Group. Effects of intensive glucose lowering in type 2 diabetes. *N Engl J Med.* 2008;358(24):2545–2559.
2. The ACCORD Study Group. Long-term effects of intensive glucose lowering on cardiovascular outcomes. *N Engl J Med.* 2011;364(9):818–828.
3. Ismail-Beigi F et al. Effect of intensive treatment of hyperglycaemia on microvascular outcomes in type 2 diabetes: an analysis of the ACCORD randomised trial. *Lancet.* 2010;376(9739):419–430.
4. Duckworth W et al. Glucose control and vascular complications in veterans with type 2 diabetes. *N Engl J Med.* 2009;360(2):129–139.

5. The ADVANCE Collaborative Group. Intensive blood glucose control and vascular outcomes in patients with type 2 diabetes. *N Engl J Med.* 2008;358(24):2560–2572.

6. American Diabetes Association. Standards of medical care in diabetes—2014. *Diabetes Care.* 2014;37(Suppl 1):S14.

7. Handelsman Y et al. American Association of Clinical Endocrinologists Medical Guidelines for Clinical Practice for developing a diabetes mellitus comprehensive care plan. *Endocr Pract.* 2011;17(Suppl 2):1.

10

Intensive versus Conventional Glycemic Control in Type 1 Diabetes Mellitus

The DCCT Trial

THOMAS KRILEY

> Intensive [insulin] therapy effectively delays the onset and slows the progression of diabetic retinopathy, nephropathy, and neuropathy in patients with [type I] diabetes mellitus.
> —DCCT RESEARCH GROUP[1]

Research Question: In patients with type I diabetes mellitus, does intensive management of blood sugar with insulin reduce the development and progression of microvascular complications from diabetes?[1]

Funding: The National Institute of Diabetes and Digestive and Kidney Diseases, the National Heart, Lung, and Blood Institute, and the National Eye Institute.

Year Study Began: 1983

Year Study Published: 1993

Study Location: 29 centers in the United States and Canada.

Who Was Studied: Patients 13–39 years old with type I diabetes mellitus. Patients with type 1 diabetes for 1 to 5 years, without evidence of retinopathy, and urinary albumin excretion <40 mg per 24 hours were included in the primary prevention cohort. Those with type 1 diabetes for 1 to 15 years, mild to moderate nonproliferative retinopathy, and urinary albumin excretion <200 mg per 24 hours were included in the secondary intervention cohort.

Who Was Excluded: Patients with concurrent hypertension, hyperlipidemia, "severe diabetic complications," or other significant medical conditions.

How Many Patients: 1,441

Study Overview: See Figure 10.1 for a summary of the DCCT's design.

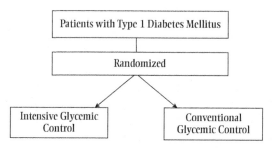

Figure 10.1 Summary of the Study Design.

Study Intervention: Patients were randomized to receive either conventional or intensive insulin therapy. Conventional therapy consisted of one to two insulin injections per day, daily glucose monitoring performed by the patient, and education on diet and exercise. The goals of conventional therapy included controlling symptoms from diabetes, prevention of ketonuria, avoidance of hypoglycemia, and maintenance of normal growth.

Intensive therapy consisted of three or more insulin injections per day or use of an insulin pump. Dosing adjustments were based on daily "self-monitoring of blood glucose [at least four measurements per day], dietary intake, and anticipated exercise." Patients had monthly follow-up appointments and regular telephone contact to review their insulin regimen. Target blood sugars were as follows: Preprandial: 70–120 mg/dl; postprandial: <180 mg/dl; a weekly 3 A.M. blood glucose >65 mg/dl; and a hemoglobin A1c of <6.05%.

Follow-Up: Mean of 6.5 years.

Endpoints: Development or progression of retinopathy on biannual fundo-scopic examination (defined as a sustained increase of three or more steps on the Early Treatment of Diabetic Retinopathy Study scale); development of severe nonproliferative or proliferative retinopathy; incidence of nephropathy, defined as the development of microalbuminuria (urinary albumin excretion ≥40 mg per 24 hours) or albuminuria (≥300 mg of albumin excretion per 24 hours); and development of neuropathy not present at baseline.

RESULTS

- Patients in the intensive therapy group had significantly lower glycosylated hemoglobin levels (~7% in the intensive therapy group versus ~9% in the conventional therapy group) and lower average blood glucose levels (155±30 mg/dl with intensive therapy versus 231±55 mg/dl with conventional therapy, $P < 0.001$).
- Patients in both the primary prevention and secondary intervention cohorts were less likely to develop microvascular complications from diabetes (Table 10.1).
- Intensive therapy was associated with a reduction in the number of patients developing hypercholesterolemia (defined as LDL>160 mg/dl, 34% risk reduction, $P = 0.02$); patients given intensive therapy also experienced a nonsignificant reduction in the number of major cardiovascular and peripheral vascular events.
- The risk of significant hypoglycemia was higher in the intensive therapy group compared to the conventional therapy group (62 versus 19 episodes per 100 patient-years).
- At 5 years, patients receiving intensive therapy had a mean weight gain of 4.6 kg (10.1 lbs) relative to the conventional therapy group.
- Quality-of-life scores were similar between the two groups throughout the trial.

Table 10.1. SUMMARY OF KEY FINDINGS

	Primary Prevention			Secondary Intervention		
	Conventional Therapy	Intensive Therapy	P Value	Conventional Therapy	Intensive Therapy	P Value
	Rate/100 patient-years			Rate/100 patient-years		
Retinopathy	4.7	1.2	≤0.002	7.8	3.7	≤0.002
Microalbuminuria	3.4	2.2	<0.04	5.7	3.6	≤0.002
Albuminuria	0.3	0.2	nonsignificant	1.4	0.6	<0.04
Neuropathy at 5 Years	9.8	3.1	<0.04	16.1	7.0	≤0.002

Criticisms and Limitations: Participants in this study were young and relatively healthy (without additional underlying medical disorders such as hypertension or hyperlipidemia), which raises concerns about the generalizability of the results. Additionally, concerns have been raised about the high number of hypoglycemic episodes experienced in the intensive therapy group.

Other Relevant Studies and Information:

- The Epidemiology of Diabetes Interventions and Complications (EDIC) study was a longitudinal, observational study that followed 93% of the patients included in the DCCT study. Patients who received intensive versus conventional therapy had a 42% risk reduction in cardiovascular disease after 17 years of follow-up.[2]
- The American Diabetes Association (ADA) recommends targeting a glycosylated hemoglobin <7% soon after diagnosis in patients with type 1 diabetes to reduce micro- and macrovascular complications. This target can be adjusted upward or downward, depending on the patient's ability to avoid episodes of hypoglycemia.[3]

Summary and Implications: Intensive glycemic management targeting preprandial blood sugars of 70–120 mg/dl and postprandial blood sugars of <180 mg/dl results in a decreased risk of microvascular complications including retinopathy, nephropathy, and neuropathy relative to conventional therapy. Follow-up analyses suggest that intensive therapy also reduces macrovascular complications. The benefits of intensive therapy must be balanced against the risk for hypoglycemia. The ADA guidelines recommend a target glycosylated hemoglobin A1c of <7% for most patients with diabetes, including those with type 1 diabetes.

CLINICAL CASE: DIABETES TREATMENT GOALS

Case History:
A 16-year-old girl presents to your clinic for hospital follow-up after being diagnosed with type 1 diabetes mellitus. The patient had been experiencing polyuria and weight loss for some time and presented to the emergency room last week in diabetic ketoacidosis. At that time the patient's blood sugar was 542 mg/dl. The patient was started on long- and short-acting insulin therapy at discharge. Based on the results of the DCCT trial, what target glycosylated

hemoglobin level is most appropriate for this patient and how should her insulin dosing be managed?

Suggested Answer:

Based on the DCCT study and the follow-up analysis, intensive blood sugar management decreases microvascular and macrovascular complications in patients with type I diabetes. This patient should receive lifestyle counseling and education on regular blood glucose monitoring and insulin adjustment. Based on the ADA guidelines, her initial target glycosylated hemoglobin should be <7% and perhaps lower if this can be achieved while avoiding hypoglycemic episodes. As this patient has a new diagnosis of type 1 diabetes, she may have some residual beta cell function, and thus she should be monitored closely for hypoglycemia, which is important for any patient who begins insulin therapy.

References

1. The Diabetes Control and Complications Trial Research Group. The effect of intensive treatment of diabetes on the development and progression of long-term complications in insulin-dependent diabetes mellitus. *N Engl J Med*. 1993;329:977.
2. Nathan D. Intensive diabetes treatment and cardiovascular disease in patients with type 1 diabetes. *N Engl J Med*. 2005 Dec 22,353(25):2643.
3. Executive summary: standards of medical care in diabetes—2014. *Diabetes Care*. 2014 Jan(Suppl 1):S5–S13.

11

Intensive versus Conservative Blood Pressure Control in Patients with Type 2 Diabetes

The ACCORD-BP Trial

STEVEN D. HOCHMAN

> The results provide no evidence that the strategy of intensive blood pressure control reduces the rate . . . of major cardiovascular events in [patients with type 2 diabetes].
>
> —THE ACCORD STUDY GROUP[1]

Research Question: In patients with type 2 diabetes, is an intensive systolic blood pressure target of <120 mm Hg better than a less aggressive target of <140 mm Hg?[1]

Funding: The National Heart, Lung, and Blood Institute and other branches of the National Institutes of Health.

Year Study Began: 2001

Year Study Published: 2010

Study Location: 77 centers in the United States and Canada.

Who Was Studied: Adults between 40 and 79 years of age with type 2 diabetes, glycosylated hemoglobin >7.5%, and known cardiovascular disease or risk factors.

Who Was Excluded: Patients with a body mass index >45, those with a creatinine >1.5 mg/dL, and those with "other serious illnesses."

How Many Patients: 4,733

Study Overview: See Figure 11.1 for a summary of the ACCORD-BP study's design.

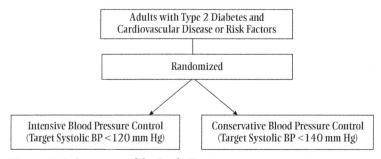

Figure 11.1 Summary of the Study Design.

Study Intervention: Patients randomized to intensive blood pressure control were prescribed antihypertensive medications to target a systolic blood pressure of <120 mm Hg. Patients in the conservative blood pressure treatment group were prescribed antihypertensive medications to target a systolic blood pressure of <140 mm Hg. For patients in the conservative treatment group, antihypertensive therapy was reduced if the systolic blood pressure was <130 mm Hg at any follow-up visit or <135 mm Hg at two consecutive visits. Patients in the intensive group had follow-up visits every 1–2 months versus every 3–4 months in the conservative group.

Follow-Up: Mean of 4.7 years.

Endpoints: Primary outcome: A composite of nonfatal myocardial infarction, nonfatal stroke, and cardiovascular mortality. Secondary outcome: All-cause mortality.

RESULTS:

- Baseline characteristics were similar between the two groups with a mean age of 62 years and a mean blood pressure of 139/76 mm Hg; 48% of participants were female and 34% had experienced a previous cardiovascular event.
- Patients in the intensive therapy group received more antihypertensive medications and had lower mean blood pressures after one year of follow-up compared to the conservative therapy group (Table 11.1).
- Except for a modest absolute reduction in the rate of stroke in the intensive therapy group, outcomes were similar between the two groups (Table 11.1).
- There was a higher rate of adverse events attributed to blood pressure medication in the intensive therapy group compared to the conservative therapy group (3.3% versus 1.3%, $P < 0.001$).

Table 11.1. SUMMARY OF KEY FINDINGS

Variable	Intensive Group	Conservative Group	P Value
Mean Blood Pressure at 1 Year	119/64	134/71	not reported
Mean Number of Antihypertensive Medications	3.4	2.1	not reported
Primary Outcome Composite	1.87%/year	2.09%/year	0.20
Nonfatal Myocardial Infarction	1.13%/year	1.28%/year	0.25
Nonfatal Stroke	0.30%/year	0.47%/year	0.03
CV Mortality	0.52%/year	0.49%/year	0.74
All-Cause Mortality	1.28%/year	1.19%/year	0.55

Criticisms and Limitations: The event rate in the conservative therapy group was half of that anticipated, perhaps due to a high rate of statin use or reduced percentage of patients with hyperlipidemia among the participants (many eligible patients with hyperlipidemia were directed to a different arm of this study, not reported here, and as a result there was a relatively low proportion of participants with hyperlipidemia in this arm). The lower-than-expected event rate may have reduced the power of the study to demonstrate significant findings.

Other Relevant Studies and Information:

- Previous trials among patients with type 2 diabetes have demonstrated the benefit of blood pressure control on microvascular complications and cardiovascular morbidity and mortality; however, in these studies less aggressive targets were used.[2,3,4] Specifically, in these trials mean blood pressure levels of 144/82, 140/81, and 135/74 were achieved in the intervention groups.
- The 2014 Evidence-Based Guideline for the Management of High Blood Pressure in Adults[5] recommends a target blood pressure <140/90 in patients with diabetes.

Summary and Implications: The ACCORD-BP trial demonstrated similar outcomes in high-risk patients with diabetes who were treated with an intensive systolic blood pressure target of <120 mm Hg versus a less aggressive target of <140 mm Hg. Although rates of stroke were lower in the intensive therapy group, adverse events from drug therapy were higher with the more intensive target. In light of these findings, guidelines recommend a blood pressure target of <140/90 mm Hg among patients with diabetes.

CLINICAL CASE: HYPERTENSION TREATMENT GOALS IN PATIENTS WITH TYPE 2 DIABETES

Case History:
A 53-year-old man with a 10-year history of type 2 diabetes treated with metformin and daily insulin injections is found on routine examination to have a blood pressure of 150/94. He is not currently on any blood pressure medications, and his previous blood pressures have always been <140/90. Laboratory studies are notable for a glycosylated hemoglobin level of 7.1%, a urinary albumin to creatinine ratio of 46 μg/mg, and a serum creatinine of 0.9 mg/dL. He returns 1 month later and his blood pressure is found to be 152/94. Based on the results of the ACCORD-BP trial, how should this patient's elevated blood pressure be managed?

Suggested Answer:
The onset of hypertension among patients with a history of diabetes is common and, if untreated, has been associated with an increased risk of cardiovascular and renal morbidity and mortality. This patient shows evidence

of moderately increased albuminuria (previously known as "microalbuminuria") and evidence of early renal disease likely caused by diabetes and hypertension. This patient should be advised that his elevated blood pressure increases his risk of developing complications from diabetes. If his blood pressure remains >140/90 in follow-up monitoring, he should be started on antihypertensive medication therapy—perhaps an angiotensin-converting enzyme (ACE) inhibitor because of his albuminuria—with a target blood pressure of <140/90. Targeting a lower blood pressure is unlikely to significantly reduce his risk for cardiovascular disease, but it may increase the risk of adverse effects related to his medications.

References

1. ACCORD Study Group et al. Effects of intensive blood-pressure control in type 2 diabetes mellitus. *N Engl J Med*. 2010;362:1575.
2. UK Prospective Diabetes Study Group. Tight blood pressure control and risk of macrovascular and microvascular complications in type 2 diabetes: UKPDS 38. *BMJ*. 1998;317:703.
3. Hansson L et al. Effects of intensive blood-pressure lowering and low-dose aspirin in patients with hypertension: principal results of the Hypertension Optimal Treatment (HOT) randomised trial. HOT Study Group. *Lancet*. 1998;351:1755.
4. Patel A et al. Effects of a fixed combination of perindopril and indapamide on macrovascular and microvascular outcomes in patients with type 2 diabetes mellitus (the ADVANCE trial): a randomised controlled trial. *Lancet*. 2007;370:829.
5. James PA et al. 2014 evidence-based guideline for the management of high blood pressure in adults: report from the panel members appointed to the Eighth Joint National Committee (JNC 8). *JAMA*. 2014;311:507.

Hematology and Oncology

12

Choice of Anticoagulant for Prevention of Recurrent Venous Thromboembolism in Patients with Cancer

The CLOT Trial

LAALITHA SURAPANENI

> Our study shows that the risk of symptomatic, recurrent thromboembolism among patients with active cancer is significantly lower with dalteparin therapy than with oral anticoagulant therapy.
>
> —LEE ET AL.[1]

Research Question: In patients with active cancer and an episode of symptomatic venous thromboembolism, is low-molecular-weight heparin (dalteparin) or oral anticoagulation with warfarin better at preventing recurrent thromboembolism?[1]

Funding: Pharmacia, the maker of dalteparin.

Year Study Began: 1999

Year Study Published: 2003

Study Location: 48 clinical centers in eight countries.

Who Was Studied: Adults with newly diagnosed, recurrent, or metastatic cancer (other than basal or squamous cell skin cancer) or cancer treatment within the last 6 months and with recently diagnosed symptomatic proximal deep vein thrombosis, pulmonary embolism, or both.

Who Was Excluded: Patients who had already received heparin or oral anticoagulants prior to enrollment. Also excluded were patients with active or recent serious bleeding, those with risk factors for serious bleeding or a platelet count less than 75,000 per cubic millimeter, patients weighing ≤40 kg, patients with a creatinine ≥3 times the upper limit of normal, and those with poor performance status (Eastern Cooperative Oncology Group performance status score of 3 or 4).

How Many Patients: 672

Study Overview: See Figure 12.1 for a summary of the study's design.

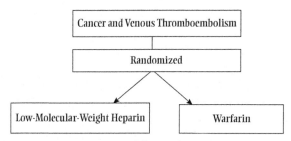

Figure 12.1 Summary of the Study Design.

Study Intervention: Patients in the warfarin group received dalteparin bridging therapy for 5–7 days followed by warfarin with dosing adjustments to target an internationalized normalized ratio of 2.5. Patients in the dalteparin group received daily injections of dalteparin 200 IU per kilogram of body weight for the first month and then approximately 150 IU per kilogram of body weight thereafter, with dosing adjustments based on platelet count. The maximum dose of dalteparin for both groups was not to exceed 18,000 IU daily.

Follow-Up: Six months.

Endpoints: Primary outcomes: Recurrent proximal deep vein thrombosis (or unequivocal extension of a preexisting thrombus), pulmonary embolism, or both. Secondary outcomes: Clinically overt bleeding and death.

RESULTS

- Baseline characteristics were similar between the two groups: 90% of study patients had solid tumors and 67% had metastatic disease at the time of enrollment.
- Recurrent thromboembolism was lower in the dalteparin group compared to the oral anticoagulant group (Table 12.1).
- There was no significant difference in bleeding events between the two groups (Table 12.1).
- There was no significant difference in mortality between the two groups (Table 12.1).

Table 12.1. Summary of Key Findings

Outcome	Oral Anticoagulant	Dalteparin	*P* Value
Recurrent Venous Thromboembolism[a]	17%	9%	0.002
Deep Vein Thrombosis	11%	4%	not reported
Pulmonary Embolism	5%	4%	not reported
Bleeding from All Causes	19%	14%	0.09
Major Bleeding[b]	4%	6%	0.27
Mortality	41%	39%	0.53

[a] Predicted rates over 6 months.
[b] Major bleeding was defined as bleeding resulting in death, occurring at a critical site (intracranial, intraspinal, intraocular, retroperitoneal, or pericardial), or bleeding resulting in the transfusion of two or more units of blood or a drop in hemoglobin of at least 2.0g/dL.

Criticisms and Limitations: This study demonstrated a reduction in the recurrence of thromboembolic disease with low-molecular-weight heparin; however, there was no reduction in mortality. Thromboembolic disease can cause bothersome symptoms, and thus it is an important endpoint. However, another important aim of treating thromboembolic disease is to prevent death. Of note, a post hoc analysis of this study demonstrated a reduction in mortality among a subset of patients who did not have metastatic disease when the trial began.[2]

In addition, the study was open-label by design to enhance safety of the participants, though this decision may have introduced bias.

Finally, since this study was published, several newer anticoagulants have been approved. Though this is not a limitation of this study, it is possible that these newer agents may prove superior to low-molecular-weight heparin for treating venous thromboembolic disease among patients with cancer. Future studies will be needed to determine this.

Other Relevant Studies and Information:

- A meta-analysis of seven randomized trials involving 1,908 patients with active cancer reported that, compared to oral vitamin K antagonists, low-molecular-weight heparin reduced the rate of recurrent venous thromboembolism (HR 0.47) but not bleeding episodes or mortality.[3] These results are consistent with this study.
- Practice guidelines from the American Society of Clinical Oncology[4] and the European Society for Medical Oncology[5] recommend that patients with cancer who have thromboembolic disease be treated with 6 months of low-molecular-weight heparin.

Summary and Implications: This large, randomized trial demonstrated that low-molecular-weight heparin reduces the risk of recurrent venous thromboembolism relative to treatment with warfarin among patients with active cancer. Though concerns remain about the high cost of low-molecular-weight heparin, this anticoagulant is the recommended first-line medication for venous thromboembolism among patients with active cancer. Future studies comparing low-molecular-weight heparin with newer anticoagulants in this population are much anticipated.

CLINICAL CASE: ANTICOAGULATION FOR VENOUS THROMBOEMBOLISM IN CANCER

Case History:
A 67-year-old woman with a history of breast cancer treated with lumpectomy and chemotherapy when she was 55 years old presents to the emergency department with a swollen, painful, and tender left leg for the past 2 days. An ultrasound of her leg shows an occlusive thrombus in the left femoral vein and proximal left popliteal vein. Following acute management of this deep vein thrombosis, what therapy should the patient be started on?

Suggested Answer:

The CLOT study showed that low-molecular-weight heparin is more efficacious than oral anticoagulant therapy with warfarin for secondary prophylaxis of venous thromboembolic disease among patients with active cancer.

The patient in this vignette has a distant history of cancer, however. Thus it is unclear whether low-molecular-weight heparin—which is more expensive than warfarin and requires self-injections—is necessary in her case. Still, her diagnosis of venous thromboembolic disease raises the possibility of the cancer's recurrence. Regardless of the initial choice of anticoagulant, she should be evaluated for cancer recurrence. If it turns out her cancer has recurred, low-molecular-weight heparin would be the recommended treatment for her thrombosis.

References

1. Lee AY et al. Low-molecular-weight heparin versus a coumarin for the prevention of recurrent venous thromboembolism in patients with cancer. *N Engl J Med.* 2003;349:146.
2. Lee AY et al. Randomized comparison of low molecular weight heparin and coumarin derivatives on the survival of patients with cancer and venous thromboembolism. *J Clin Oncol.* 2005 Apr 1;23(10):2123–2129.
3. Akl EA et al. Anticoagulation for the long-term treatment of venous thromboembolism in patients with cancer. *Cochrane Database Syst Rev.* 2011:CD006650.
4. Lyman GH et al. American Society of Clinical Oncology Guideline: Recommendation for venous thromboembolism prophylaxis and treatment in patients with cancer. *J Clin Onc.* 2007;25(34):5490–5505.
5. Mandala M et al. Management of venous thromboembolism (VTE) in cancer patients: ESMO Clinical Practice Guidelines. *Annals Oncol.* 2011;22 (Suppl 6):vi85–92.

13

Vena Cava Filters in the Prevention of Pulmonary Embolism in Patients with Proximal Deep Vein Thrombosis

LAALITHA SURAPANENI

> Because of the observed excess of recurrent deep vein thrombosis and the absence of any effect on mortality . . . systematic use [of vena cava filters] cannot be recommended [among patients with deep vein thrombosis at high risk for pulmonary embolism].
>
> —DECOUSUS ET AL.[1]

Research Question: Are vena cava filters, in addition to standard anticoagulation therapy, beneficial in patients with an episode of deep vein thrombosis (DVT) who are at high risk for pulmonary embolism?[1]

Funding: Rhône-Poulenc (now a part of Sanofi), makers of enoxaparin, as well as the French Ministry of Health and French Health Insurance Fund.

Year Study Began: 1991

Year Study Published: 1998

Study Location: 44 centers in France.

Who Was Studied: Adult patients with acute proximal DVT confirmed by venography whose physicians considered them to be at high risk for pulmonary embolism. Patients were included if they presented with or without concomitant pulmonary embolism.

Who Was Excluded: Patients who had a history of, or contraindication to, vena cava filter placement or a contraindication to anticoagulation. Also excluded were those in need of thrombolysis and those with kidney or liver disease, or other conditions thought to limit survival. Pregnant women were also excluded.

How Many Patients: 400

Study Overview: See Figure 13.1 for a summary of the study design.

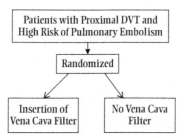

Figure 13.1 Summary of the Study Design.

Study Intervention: Patients in both groups were started on anticoagulation (either unfractionated heparin or low-molecular-weight heparin). On day 4 of anticoagulation therapy, patients were transitioned to an oral anticoagulant (either warfarin or acenocoumarol), and anticoagulation therapy was continued for at least 3 months.

Patients assigned to the vena cava filter group received one of four types of non-removable filters, which were inserted via the femoral or jugular vein under fluoroscopic guidance. Patients in the control group did not undergo filter placement.

All patients underwent a ventilation-perfusion scan within 2 days of randomization to detect the presence of pulmonary emboli at baseline. Patients with clinically suspected pulmonary embolism during the first 12 days of follow-up were assessed for pulmonary embolus with ventilation-perfusion scanning, and all remaining patients were assessed with a ventilation-perfusion scan between days 8 and 12 to diagnose asymptomatic pulmonary emboli. Diagnosis of pulmonary embolism by abnormal ventilation-perfusion scans was confirmed with pulmonary angiography. After 12 days of follow-up, patients and their general practitioners were asked to report recurrent DVT or pulmonary embolism, and at 2 years all patients were contacted by telephone and questioned about the occurrence of thromboembolic or hemorrhagic events.

Follow-up: 2 years.

Endpoints: Primary outcome: Pulmonary embolism, symptomatic or asymptomatic, within 12 days of randomization. Secondary outcomes: Recurrent DVT, death, major filter complications, and major bleeding.

RESULTS

- Baseline characteristics between the groups were similar with an average age of 73 years; 48% of patients were male.
- At baseline, 49% of patients had a pulmonary embolism, and of these 74% were symptomatic.
- In the vena cava filter group, 2% of patients did not receive a filter, and 4% of patients in the non–vena cava filter group had a filter placed.
- By day 12, patients in the filter group experienced fewer pulmonary emboli compared to the control group (Table 13.1).
- After 2 years, patients in the filter group experienced higher rates of DVT compared to the control group (Table 13.1); in the filter group, 43% of these DVTs occurred at the filter sites.
- There were no differences between the groups in mortality, symptomatic pulmonary embolism, or major bleeding at 2 years (Table 13.1).

Table 13.1. SUMMARY OF KEY FINDINGS

Outcome	Vena Cava Filter	No Vena Cava Filter	*P* Value
At Day 12			
Symptomatic Pulmonary Embolism	1%	3%	not reported
Asymptomatic Pulmonary Embolism	0%	2%	not reported
Total Pulmonary Embolism	1%	5%	0.03
At 2 Years			
Symptomatic Pulmonary Embolism	3%	6%	0.16
Recurrent DVT	21%	12%	0.02
Major Bleeding	9%	12%	0.41
Mortality	22%	20%	0.65

Criticisms and Limitations: Retrospective calculations suggest that this study was underpowered to detect significant differences in symptomatic pulmonary embolism and mortality between the groups. In addition, subjective inclusion criteria were used to select patients for this study (i.e., their physicians felt they were at high risk for pulmonary embolism). It is possible that vena cava filter placement would prove beneficial among a carefully selected subset of patients. Finally, it is notable that patients with contraindications to anticoagulant therapy were excluded from this study, and thus these results do not apply to such patients.

Other Relevant Studies and Information:

- An 8-year follow-up analysis of this study revealed that patients who underwent filter placement had higher rates of DVT (35% versus 27%), lower rates of pulmonary embolism (1% versus 5%), and similar rates of overall mortality.[2]
- There are few other high-quality studies evaluating the effectiveness of vena cava filters, and there are no other high-quality randomized trials.[3]
- The American College of Chest Physician guidelines recommend against the use of vena cava filters in cases of acute DVT or pulmonary embolism unless there is a contraindication to anticoagulation such as recent surgery or hemorrhagic stroke.[4] Data suggest that these guidelines are frequently disregarded, however.[5]

Summary and Implications: For patients with proximal DVT at high risk for pulmonary embolism, placing an inferior vena cava filter in addition to standard anticoagulation therapy reduces the risk of pulmonary embolism but increases the risk of recurrent DVT and does not reduce mortality.

CLINICAL CASE: PLACEMENT OF INFERIOR VENA CAVA FILTER FOR DVT

Case History:

A 64-year-old man with a past medical history of stage III squamous cell lung carcinoma presents with a swollen, painful right leg. Ultrasonography reveals a partially occlusive thrombus in the right femoral vein. He is started on anticoagulation therapy with low-molecular-weight heparin. Given his history of malignancy, he is deemed to be at high risk for venous thromboembolic events and development of a pulmonary embolism.

Based on the results of this study, would this patient benefit from the addition of an inferior vena cava filter?

Suggested Answer:

This patient presents with acute DVT and a high risk for recurrent thrombosis and development of pulmonary embolism. He should be treated with anticoagulation therapy—ideally low-molecular-weight heparin[6]—for at least three months. Placement of an inferior vena cava filter may reduce the risk of pulmonary embolism in the first 12 days; however, it would increase his risk of recurrent DVT and is unlikely to improve his survival. Thus, he should not receive a filter.

References

1. Decousus H et al. A clinical trial of vena caval filters in the prevention of pulmonary embolism in patients with proximal DVT. *N Engl J Med*. 1998;338:409–415.
2. PREPIC Study Group. Eight-year follow-up of patients with permanent vena cava filters in the prevention of pulmonary embolism: the PREPIC (Prevention du Risque d'Embolie Pulmonaire par Interruption Cave) randomized study. *Circulation*. 2005;112:416.
3. Girard P, Stern JB, Parent F. Medical literature and vena cava filters: so far so weak. *Chest*. 2002;122(3):963.
4. Guyatt GH et al. Antithrombotic therapy and prevention of thrombosis (9th edition): American College of Chest Physicians evidence-based clinical practice guidelines. *Chest*. 2012;141:7S–47S.
5. White RH et al. High variation between hospitals in vena cava filter use for venous thromboembolism. *JAMA Intern Med*. 2013 Apr;173(7):506–512.
6. Lee AY et al. Low-molecular-weight heparin versus a coumarin for the prevention of recurrent venous thromboembolism in patients with cancer. *N Engl J Med*. 2003;349(2):146.

14

Phase I Study of Imatinib (STI571) in Patients with Chronic Myeloid Leukemia

JOSHUA R. THOMAS

STI571 (imatinib) is well tolerated and has significant antileukemic activity in patients with [chronic myeloid leukemia] in whom treatment with interferon alfa had failed.

—DRUKER ET AL.[1]

Research Question: Is imatinib (STI571)—a compound developed to target a mutant protein in chronic myeloid leukemia (CML) cells—safe and effective for the treatment of CML?[1]

Funding: The National Cancer Institute, the Leukemia and Lymphoma Society, and Novartis Pharmaceuticals, the maker of imatinib (Gleevec).

Year Study Began: 1998

Year Study Published: 2001

Study Location: Three centers in the United States.

Who Was Studied: Adults with CML who tested positive for the Philadelphia chromosome (a translocation that results in the generation of an oncogenic fusion protein known as BCR-ABL, which is targeted by imatinib). Patients were eligible if they were in the chronic phase of CML (<15% blasts or baso-phils in the peripheral blood or bone marrow) and were resistant to or were intolerant of treatment with interferon alfa.

Who Was Excluded: Patients with a platelet count of <100,000/mL³ and those with substantial renal, hepatic, or cardiac impairment or low-performance status.

How Many Patients: 83

Study Overview: See Figure 14.1 for a summary of the study's design.

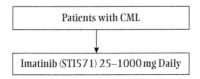

*Note that this was a phase I study and there was no control group.

Figure 14.1 Summary of the Study Design.

Study Intervention: All patients were treated with imatinib by mouth 1–2 times daily with a total daily dose ranging from 25–1000 mg. This was a dose-escalation trial, and consecutive cohorts of enrolled patients were started on imatinib at increasing doses (e.g., cohort 1 started on 25 mg daily, cohort 2 started on 50 mg daily, etc.).

Follow-Up: The median duration of treatment was 310 days (a range of 17 to 607 days).

Endpoints: Primary outcome: Safety and tolerability. Secondary outcomes: Partial or complete hematologic response to therapy. A partial response was defined as a ≥50% reduction in the white blood cell count from baseline maintained for at least 2 weeks. A complete response was defined as a reduction in the white blood cell count to <10,000 and a reduction in the platelet count to <450,000 maintained for 4 weeks. In addition, patients were assessed for a cytogenetic response with bone marrow biopsies to assess the percentage of cells positive for the Philadelphia chromosome during metaphase (0% = complete response; 1%–35% = partial response; 36%–65% = minor response; and >65% = absent response).

RESULTS

- The median age of participants was 55 years and 66% were male; the median duration of disease at the time of enrollment was 3.8 years with a median white blood cell count and platelet count of 27,800 cells/mm^3 and 430,000 cells/mm^3, respectively.
- STI571 was well tolerated with nausea, myalgias, edema, and diarrhea being the most common side effects; most side effects, even at high doses, were graded as mild to moderate.
- At least a partial hematologic response was achieved in all patients treated with 140 mg or more, and a complete hematologic response occurred in 53 of 54 patients treated with ≥300 mg.
- A cytogenetic response to therapy occurred in 54% of patients taking ≥300 mg of the study medication, and of those with a cytogenic response, 59% had a complete or partial response and 41% had a minor response.

Criticisms and Limitations: The study did not follow patients beyond 1 year and did not assess hard outcomes such as survival rates, though such outcomes are not the focus of phase I trials. In addition, because this was a phase I dose escalation trial, there was no control group.

Other Relevant Studies and Information:

- The IRIS trial randomized 1,106 patients with chronic CML to imatinib or interferon alpha plus cytarabine and found superior hematologic and cytogenetic responses, decreased progression of CML to advanced stages of disease, and higher medication tolerability with imatinib.[2]
- The second-generation tyrosine kinase inhibitors dasatinib and nilotinib have been compared to imatinib in randomized trials showing faster responses to therapy and a higher proportion of patients with a complete cytogenetic response.[3,4]
- A third-generation tyrosine kinase inhibitor, ponatinib, developed in response to cancers resistant to first- and second-generation tyrosine kinase inhibitors, has demonstrated high efficacy in early phase trials.[5]
- The National Comprehensive Cancer Network guidelines recommend initial treatment of CML patients with positive results for the Philadelphia chromosome with imatinib, dasatinib, or nilotinib.[6]

Summary and Implications: This study was the first to demonstrate the efficacy of targeted therapy against CML cells with the Philadelphia chromosome translocation. Because of this and subsequent studies, imatinib and related therapies have become the standard of care for patients with CML. The development of these targeted therapies is also significant because it represents one of the first successful instances of systematic drug development aimed at targeting specific cancer mutations.

CLINICAL CASE: TARGETED THERAPY IN CML

Case History:

A 54-year-old man is evaluated in the hospital for increasing fatigue for the past 2 months. He has a history of hypertension, dyslipidemia, and diabetes treated with lisinopril, simvastatin, and metformin. His vital signs are within normal limits and there is no lymphadenopathy or edema on physical examination. The spleen is palpable 3 cm below the left costal margin. Labs show a hemoglobin of 11.9 g/dL with a white blood cell count of 54,300/μL, and a platelet count of 120,000/μL. A peripheral blood smear shows an increased number of granulocytic cells. A bone marrow aspiration is performed and significant granulocytosis is noted. Cytogenetic studies are positive for the Philadelphia chromosome.

Based on the results of this trial, how should this patient be treated?

Suggested Answer:

This patient should be referred to a hematologist or oncologist and started on imatinib (STI571) or another related tyrosine kinase inhibitor as his first-line therapy.

References

1. Druker BJ et al. Efficacy and safety of a specific inhibitor of the BCR-ABL tyrosine kinase in chronic myeloid leukemia. *N Engl J Med.* 2001;344:1031.
2. O'Brien SG et al. Imatinib compared with interferon and low-dose cytarabine for newly diagnosed chronic-phase chronic myeloid leukemia. *N Engl J Med.* 2003;348:994.
3. Saglio G et al. Nilotinib versus imatinib for newly diagnosed chronic myeloid leukemia. *N Engl J Med.* 2010;362:2251.

4. Kantarjian H et al. Dasatinib versus imatinib in newly diagnosed chronic-phase chronic myeloid leukemia. *N Engl J Med*. 2010;362:2260.

5. Cortes JE et al. A phase 2 trial of ponatinib in Philadelphia chromosome–positive leukemias. *N Engl J Med*. 2013;369:1783–1796.

6. O'Brien S et al. NCCN clinical practice guidelines in oncology: chronic myelogenous leukemia. *J Natl Compr Canc Netw*. 2009;7(9):984–1023.

SECTION 4

Musculoskeletal Diseases

15

Magnetic Resonance Imaging for Low Back Pain

MICHAEL E. HOCHMAN

Although . . . patients preferred [rapid MRI scans to plain radiographs for the evaluation of low back pain], substituting rapid MRI for radiographic evaluations . . . may offer little additional benefit to patients, and it may increase the costs of care because of the increased number of spine operations that patients are likely to undergo.

—JARVIK ET AL.[1]

Research Question: Should patients with low back pain requiring imaging be offered plain radiographs or magnetic resonance imaging (MRI)?[1]

Funding: The Agency for Healthcare Research and Quality, and the National Institute for Arthritis and Musculoskeletal and Skin Diseases.

Year Study Began: 1998

Year Study Published: 2003

Study Location: Four imaging sites in Washington State (an outpatient clinic, a teaching hospital, a multispecialty clinic, and a private imaging center).

Who Was Studied: Adults 18 years of age and older referred by their physician for radiographs of the lumbar spine to evaluate lower back pain and/or radiculopathy.

Who Was Excluded: Patients with lumbar surgery within the previous year, those with acute external trauma, and those with metallic implants in the spine.

How Many Patients: 380

Study Overview: See Figure 15.1 for a summary of the study design.

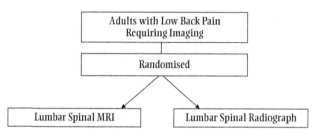

Figure 15.1 Summary of the Study Design.

Study Intervention: Patients assigned to the plain radiograph group received the films according to standard protocol. Most patients received anteroposterior and lateral views only. However, a small number received additional views when requested by the ordering physician.

Patients assigned to the MRI group were scheduled for the scan on the day of study enrollment whenever possible, and if not within a week of enrollment. Most scans were performed with a field strength of 1.5 T, and all patients received sagittal and axial T2-weighted images.

Follow-Up: 12 months.

Endpoints: Primary outcome: Scores on the 23-item modified Roland-Morris back pain disability scale.[2] Secondary outcomes: Quality of life as assessed using the Medical Outcomes Study 36-Item Short Form Survey (SF-36);[3] patient satisfaction with care as assessed using the Deyo-Diehl patient satisfaction questionnaire;[4] days of lost work; patient reassurance; and health care resource utilization.

The 23-item modified Roland-Morris back pain disability scale consists of 23 "yes" or "no" questions. Patients are given one point for each "yes" answer for a total possible score of 23. Below are sample questions on the scale:

- I stay at home most of the time because of my back problem or leg pain (sciatica)

- I walk more slowly than usual because of my back problem or leg pain (sciatica)
- I stay in bed most of the time because of my back or leg pain (sciatica)

RESULTS

- The mean age of study patients was 53; 15% were either unemployed, disabled, or on leave from work; 24% had depression; and 70% reported pain radiating to the legs.
- 49% of patients were referred for imaging by primary care doctors, while 51% were referred by specialists.
- The spinal MRI revealed disk herniation in 33% of patients, nerve root impingement in 7%, moderate or severe central canal stenosis in 20%, and lateral recess stenosis in 17%—findings that are typically not detectable with plain radiographs.
- There were no significant differences in back pain scores between the radiograph and MRI groups though patients in the MRI group were more likely to be reassured by their imaging results; there were no significant differences in total health care costs between the groups (see Tables 15.1 and 15.2).

Table 15.1. Summary of Key Findings[a]

Outcome	Radiograph Group	MRI Group	P Value
Roland-Morris Back Pain Score (Scale: 0–23)[b]	8.75	9.34	0.53
SF-36, Physical Functioning (Scale: 0–100)[c]	63.77	61.04	not significant[d]
Patient Satisfaction (Scale: 0–11)[c]	7.34	7.04	not significant[d]
Days of Lost Work in Past 4 Weeks	1.26	1.57	not significant[d]
Were you reassured by the imaging results?	58%	74%	0.002

[a] The 12-month outcomes were adjusted for baseline scores. For example, the 12-month Roland scores were adjusted for the fact that, at baseline, scores were slightly higher in patients randomized to the MRI group.
[b] Higher scores indicate a worse outcome.
[c] Higher scores indicate a better outcome.
[d] Actual P value not reported.

Table 15.2. COMPARISON OF RESOURCE UTILIZATION DURING
THE STUDY PERIOD

Outcome	Radiograph Group	MRI Group	*P* Value
Patients Receiving Opioid Analgesics	25%	26%	0.94
Subsequent MRIs per Patient	0.22	0.09	0.01
Physical Therapy, Acupuncture, and Massage Visits per Patient	7.9	3.8	0.008
Specialist Consultations per Patient	0.49	0.73	0.07
Patients Receiving Lumbar Spine Surgery	2%	6%	0.09
Total Costs of Health Care Services	$1,651	$2,121	0.11

Criticisms and Limitations: The increased rate of spinal surgeries and the higher cost of health care services in the MRI group did not reach statistical significance. Therefore, it is not appropriate to draw firm conclusions from these findings.

Other Relevant Studies and Information:

- Other trials have suggested that early spinal imaging (radiographs, computed tomography, and MRI) does not improve outcomes in patients with acute lower back pain without alarm symptoms such as worsening neurologic function,[5] nor does it substantially assist with decision making in patients referred for epidural steroid injections of the spine.[6]
- Guidelines[7] recommend that MRIs of the lumbar spine only be obtained in patients with signs or symptoms of:

  - emergent conditions such as the cauda equina syndrome, tumors, infections, or fractures with neurologic impingement
  - radicular symptoms severe enough and long-lasting enough to warrant surgical intervention
  - spinal stenosis severe enough and long-lasting enough to warrant surgical intervention.

Summary and Implications: Although spinal MRIs (compared with plain radiographs) are reassuring for patients with low back pain, they do not lead to improved functional outcomes. In addition, spinal MRIs detect anatomical abnormalities that would otherwise go undiscovered, possibly leading to spinal surgeries of uncertain value.

CLINICAL CASE: MRI FOR LOW BACK PAIN

Case History:

A 52-year-old man with 6 weeks of low back pain visits your office requesting an MRI of his spine. His symptoms began after doing yard work and have improved only slightly during this time period. The pain is bothersome, but not incapacitating, and radiates down his right leg. He has no systemic symptoms (fevers, chills, or weight loss) and denies bowel or bladder dysfunction. He reports difficulty walking due to the pain. On exam, he is an overweight man in no apparent distress. His range of motion is limited due to pain. He has no neurological deficits.

Based on the results of this trial, should you order an MRI for this patient?

Suggested Answer:

Based on the results of this trial, ordering a spinal MRI in a patient like the one in this vignette is unlikely to lead to improved functional outcomes and may increase the likelihood of spinal surgery by detecting anatomical abnormalities that would otherwise go undiscovered. Still, this trial showed that an MRI may provide reassurance to patients. For this reason, you should reassure your patient in other ways, for example, by telling him that he does not have any signs or symptoms of a serious back problem like an infection or cancer.

Other types of spinal imaging such as plain radiographs do not appear to improve outcomes in patients with acute low back pain without alarm symptoms either. Thus, even a plain film may not be necessary at this time.

References

1. Jarvik JG et al. Rapid magnetic resonance imaging vs. radiographs for patients with low back pain: a randomized controlled trial. *JAMA*. 2003;289(21):2810–2818.
2. Roland M, Morris R. A study of the natural history of back pain, 1: development of a reliable and sensitive measure of disability in low back pain. *Spine*. 1983;8:141–144.
3. Ware JE, Sherbourne CD. The MOS 36-item short-form survey (SF-36), I: conceptual framework and item selection. *Med Care*. 1992;30:473–483.
4. Deyo RA, Diehl AK. Patient satisfaction with medical care for low-back pain. *Spine*. 1986;11:28–30.
5. Chou R et al. Imaging strategies for low-back pain: systematic review and meta-analysis. *Lancet*. 2009;373(9662):463.

6. Cohen SP et al. Effect of MRI on treatment results or decision making in patients with lumbosacral radiculopathy referred for epidural steroid injections: a multi-center, randomized controlled trial. *Arch Intern Med.* 2012;172(2):134.

7. Bigos SJ et al. *Acute low back pain problems in adults.* Clinical practice guideline No 14. Rockville, MD: Agency for Health Care Policy and Research, Public Health Service, US Department of Health and Human Services, December 1994.

16

Early Therapy for Rheumatoid Arthritis

The TICORA Study

KATHRYN WHITE

> Our evidence lends support to the hypothesis that tight control [with a strategy of intensive treatment] can be achieved in most patients with early rheumatoid arthritis.
>
> —THE TICORA STUDY[1]

Research Question: Does treating rheumatoid arthritis early and aggressively prevent disease progression and improve quality of life?[1]

Funding: The Chief Scientist's Office of the Scottish Executive Health Department, an agency within the United Kingdom's National Health Service.

Year Study Began: 1999

Year Study Published: 2004

Study Location: Two academic hospitals in Glasgow, UK.

Who Was Studied: Adults between the ages of 18 and 75 with rheumatoid arthritis for fewer than 5 years and a disease activity score (DAS) >2.4. The DAS is calculated from the erythrocyte sedimentation rate, a global assessment of disease activity, and physical examination for tenderness and swelling of joints. Scores of >3.6, >2.4, and >1.6 represent high, moderate, and low disease activity, respectively. Since publication of this study, the DAS has been modified to examine

28 instead of 66 joints and is now referred to as the DAS28, in which scores of 2.6–3.2, 3.2–5.1, and >5.1 represent low, moderate, and high disease activity.

Who Was Excluded: Patients who had received combination disease-modifying antirheumatic drug treatment (DMARD) and those with laboratory evidence of liver, renal, or hematologic disease.

How Many Patients: 111

Study Overview: See Figure 16.1 for a summary of the study's design.

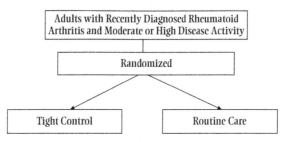

Figure 16.1 Summary of the Study Design.

Study Intervention: Participants in the tight control group were assessed monthly throughout the study. At each visit the patient's DAS was calculated and any swollen joints amenable to intra-articular steroid injections were injected. Patients in whom the DAS remained >2.4 after 3 months received an escalation of oral treatment following a stepwise protocol (Table 16.1).

Table 16.1. PROTOCOL FOR DMARD THERAPY[1]

Step 1	• Sulfasalazine 500 mg daily, increasing weekly to a target dose of 40 mg/kg/day
Step 2	• Continue sulfasalazine • Initiate methotrexate 7.5 mg weekly with folic acid 5 mg weekly • Initiate hydroxychloroquine 200–400 mg daily (maximum 6.5 mg/kg/day)
Step 3	• Continue sulfasalazine • Increase methotrexate by 2.5-5 mg monthly (maximum 25 mg weekly) • Continue hydroxychloroquine
Step 4	• Increase sulfasalazine by 500 mg weekly (maximum 5000 mg daily) • Continue methotrexate • Continue hydroxychloroquine
Step 5	• Continue triple therapy • Add prednisolone in enteric-coated tablets 7.5 mg daily
Step 6	Change triple therapy to: • Ciclosporin 2–5 mg/kg/day • Methotrexate 25 mg weekly with folic acid 5 mg weekly
Step 7	• Change to alternative disease-modifying antirheumatic therapy (leflunomide or sodium aurothiomalate)

Participants in the routine care group were assessed every 3 months in a general rheumatology clinic. Treatment was not guided by formal DAS calculation or a set protocol. Monotherapy with DMARDs was given if participants had active synovitis. Intra-articular steroid injections could be given utilizing the same protocol as in the tight control group. In cases of treatment failure ("lack of effect or toxic effects of medication"), alternative or additional DMARDs could be used at the discretion of the treating physician.

Follow-Up: 18 months.

Endpoints: Primary outcomes: A mean change in DAS, and the proportion of participants with a good response to therapy, defined as a DAS <2.4 at the end of follow-up and a fall in the DAS of at least 1.2 from the baseline. Secondary outcomes: Proportion of patients in remission at the end of follow-up (DAS <1.6), and resource utilization.

RESULTS

- Baseline characteristics were similar in both groups with an average baseline DAS of 4.9 in the tight control group versus 4.6 in the routine care group; 70% of participants were female and the average age was 53 years.
- More patients in the tight control group were prescribed combination DMARD therapy (67% versus 11%).
- DMARD therapy was discontinued due to toxic side effects more frequently in the routine versus tight control group (43% versus 16%).
- Patients in the tight control group received higher mean doses of intramuscular and intra-articular triamcinolone acetonide than those in the routine care group (28 mg/month versus 8 mg/month).
- The mean fall in DAS and proportion of patients with a good response or remission to therapy were higher in the tight control group (Table 16.2).
- The overall cost of care was lower in the tight control versus routine care group because of higher inpatient costs in the routine care group; this was despite higher costs in outpatient visits, prescribing, travel, and diagnostic testing in the tight control group.

Table 16.2. SUMMARY OF KEY FINDINGS

Variable	Tight Control Group	Routine Care Group	P Value
Change in DAS	−3.5	−1.9	<0.0001
Good Response to Treatment	82%	44%	<0.0001
Remission	65%	16%	<0.0001

Criticisms and Limitations: The multifaceted approach to therapy in the tight control group makes it difficult to determine which components of the intervention protocol led to the observed benefit.

Additionally, it appears that patients assigned to the tight control group received more attentive care than those in the routine care group. For example, patients in the tight control group received more steroid injections and were less likely to discontinue DMARD therapy due to side effects (perhaps because their physicians were more likely to encourage them to continue DMARD therapy despite mild side effects). It is thus possible that the better outcomes observed in the tight control group resulted from the more attentive care they received rather than the actual treatment protocol.

Finally, the study did not investigate the role of biologic agents in the treatment of early rheumatoid arthritis.

Other Relevant Studies and Information:

- A meta-analysis of six trials comparing tight control to usual care found a significantly greater reduction in DAS with tight control versus usual care.[2] In these trials, protocol-driven tight control therapy was more effective than non-protocol-driven tight control therapy.
- Studies have also suggested a benefit of combining biologic agents with DMARD therapy;[3] however, results from these studies have conflicted.
- The American College of Rheumatology recommends immediate treatment with DMARDs for all patients with rheumatoid arthritis with a goal of inducing disease remission or low disease activity.[4] The guidelines recommend combination therapy for patients with poor prognostic factors including extra-articular disease, positive rheumatoid factor or anti-cyclic citrullinated peptide antibodies, or bony erosions on radiographs. The guidelines also recommend consideration of biologic therapy for patients with high disease activity and poor prognostic factors.

Summary and Implications: The TICORA trial demonstrated the benefits of early tight control of rheumatoid arthritis using DMARD therapy, frequent follow-up visits, and liberal use of intra-articular steroid injections. Patients using this approach had greater reductions in disease activity and lower overall costs (because of a reduction in the need for inpatient care). The American College of Rheumatology recommends immediate DMARD therapy for all patients with rheumatoid arthritis with a goal of inducing disease remission or low disease activity.

CLINICAL CASE: INTENSIVE TREATMENT IN EARLY RHEUMATOID ARTHRITIS

Case History:

A 27-year-old woman diagnosed with rheumatoid arthritis 1 month ago and started on methotrexate presents for a follow-up visit. She has evidence of synovitis on exam but is concerned about adding a second medication and causing increased risk for side effects. Based on the TICORA study and related studies, what do you recommend?

Suggested Answer:

This patient with newly diagnosed rheumatoid arthritis has evidence of active disease despite monotherapy with methotrexate. The TICORA study demonstrated the benefits of tight control in early rheumatoid arthritis, and guidelines recommend titration of therapy to achieve disease remission or low disease activity. Because this patient is hesitant to add a second medication, you might explain to her the evidence indicating better outcomes with an early tight control therapy approach. Though DMARDs do have side effects, the benefits appear to outweigh risks. Thus, you should encourage her to begin combination therapy. If she remains hesitant, you might consider increasing the dose of methotrexate rather than adding another medication. She should continue monthly follow-up visits with intra-articular steroid injections in inflamed joints and oral therapy escalations to achieve low disease activity or remission.

References

1. Grigor C et al. Effect of a treatment strategy of tight control for rheumatoid arthritis (the TICORA study): a single-blind randomised controlled trial. *Lancet.* 2004 Jul 17–23;364(9430);263–269.
2. Schipper LG et al. Meta-analysis of tight control strategies in rheumatoid arthritis: protocolized treatment has additional value with respect to the clinical outcome. *Rheumatology* (Oxford) 2010;49:2154.
3. Goekoop-Ruiterman YP et al. Clinical and radiographic outcomes of four different treatment strategies in patients with early rheumatoid arthritis. *Arthritis Rheum.* 2005;58(2 Suppl):S126–S135.
4. Singh JA et al. 2012 update of the 2008 American College of Rheumatology recommendations for the use of disease-modifying antirheumatic drugs and biologic agents in the treatment of rheumatoid arthritis. *Arthritis Care Res.* 2012;64:625.

Nephrology

17

Revascularization versus Medical Therapy for Renal Artery Stenosis

The ASTRAL Trial

STEVEN D. HOCHMAN

> We found no evidence of a worthwhile clinical benefit after revascularization in patients with atherosclerotic renal artery stenosis.
> —ASTRAL INVESTIGATORS[1]

Research Question: Should patients with renal artery stenosis be treated with revascularization or medical therapy?[1]

Funding: The Medical Research Council of the United Kingdom, a publicly funded agency; the charity Kidney Research UK; and Medtronic, the manufacturer of the stents used in the study.

Year Study Began: 2000

Year Study Published: 2009

Study Location: 53 hospitals in the United Kingdom, 3 in Australia, and 1 in New Zealand.

Who Was Studied: Adult patients with clinical signs of atherosclerotic reno-vascular disease (e.g., "uncontrolled or refractory hypertension or unexplained renal dysfunction") were screened with renal artery imaging. Those found to have "substantial atherosclerotic stenosis in at least one renal artery"[1] were eligible for enrollment.

Who Was Excluded: Patients with a history of renal artery revascularization or planned revascularization, and those likely to require a revascularization within 6 months. Those with nonatheromatous cardiovascular disease were also excluded. In addition, patients were excluded if the treating physician felt that either revascularization or medical management was clearly indicated.

How Many Patients: 806

Study Overview: See Figure 17.1 for a summary of the study's design.

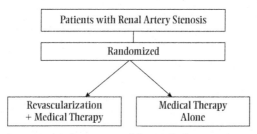

Figure 17.1 Summary of the Study Design.

Study Intervention: Patients randomized to the revascularization group received renal artery revascularization as soon as possible. Revascularization was accomplished with "angioplasty either alone or with stenting" at the discretion of the treating physician. Patients in both groups were medically managed with statins, antiplatelet agents, and antihypertensives at the discretion of the treating physician and "according to local protocols."

Follow-Up: Planned for 5 years; the median follow-up was 33.6 months.

Endpoints: Primary outcome: Change in renal function. Secondary outcomes: Blood pressure control; all-cause mortality; time to first renal event (including new onset acute kidney injury, initiation of dialysis, renal transplant, nephrectomy, or death from renal failure); time to first cardiovascular event (including myocardial infarction; hospitalization for angina, stroke, coronary or peripheral artery revascularization procedure; fluid overload or cardiac failure, or death from cardiovascular causes).

RESULTS

- At baseline, 59% of patients had >70% stenosis of at least one renal artery, and 60% had a serum creatinine >1.7 mg/dL; the estimated glomerular filtration rate (eGFR) was <50 μmol/L for 75% of patients.
- In the revascularization group, 79% of patients received a successful revascularization procedure at a median of 32 days following randomization; 6% of patients in the medical therapy group crossed over and underwent revascularization at a median of 601 days following randomization.
- There were no statistically significant differences in the change in renal function between the two groups in the intention-to-treat or per-protocol analyses (Table 17.1); subgroup analyses based on serum creatinine level, severity of stenosis, kidney length, and rate of disease progression did not yield any significant trends (i.e., it did not appear that revascularization was beneficial among any subgroups).
- Blood pressure improved in both groups with no between-group differences, though patients in the medical therapy group received slightly more antihypertensives compared to those in the revascularization group (2.97 versus 2.77, $P = 0.03$).
- There were no between-group differences in the risk of renal events, cardiovascular events, or all-cause mortality (Table 17.1).
- For patients who underwent revascularization, 9% experienced an adverse event within 24 hours of the procedure; half of these events were considered serious complications.

Table 17.1 SUMMARY OF KEY FINDINGS

Variable	Revascularization	Medical Therapy	P Value
Renal Function			
Change in Reciprocal of Creatinine[a]	$-0.07*10^{-3}$ L/μmol/yr	$-0.13*10^{-3}$ L/μmol/yr	0.06
Change in Creatinine[b]	+7.47 μmol/liter/yr	+10.52 μmol/liter/yr	
Total Renal Events	22%	22%	0.97
Acute Kidney Injury	7%	6%	not reported
End-Stage Renal Disease	8%	8%	not reported
Cardiovascular Events	49%	51%	0.96
Overall Survival	60%	57%	0.46

[a] Change in reciprocal of creatinine is assessed because it has a linear relationship with the estimated GFR. Large negative values of this variable indicate a greater worsening of renal function (i.e., renal function decreased nonsignificantly faster in the medical therapy group).
[b] Large positive values of this variable indicate a greater worsening of renal function (i.e., renal function decreased nonsignificantly faster in the medical therapy group).

Criticisms and Limitations: Patients were excluded from the study if their treating physician felt that renal artery revascularization was clearly indicated. Thus, there may have been a selection bias such that patients less likely to benefit from revascularization were disproportionately included in the study. However, there is no evidence that treating physicians can successfully select which patients are likely to benefit from renal artery revascularization.

Additionally, 41% of enrolled patients had a renal artery stenosis <70%, which may not be severe enough to cause complications such as hypertension or renal dysfunction. It is possible that the results of ASTRAL would have been different had more patients with severe stenosis been included. However, a post hoc analysis of this study and subsequent studies involving patients with more severe stenosis have also failed to demonstrate a benefit with revascularization (see the following section).

Other Relevant Studies and Information:

- Observational studies have demonstrated improvements in mortality, renal disease progression, and blood pressure control in patients selected to undergo renal artery revascularization based on specific clinical indications such as refractory hypertension, flash pulmonary edema, resistance to ACE inhibitors, or refractory heart failure.[2,3]

However, because patients in these studies were not randomized, the results are inconclusive.

- Other major randomized trials of renal artery revascularization are consistent with ASTRAL. Most notably, the CORAL trial randomized 947 patients with severe renal artery stenosis (>80% stenosis or >60% stenosis with a systolic pressure gradient of >20 mm Hg) plus either refractory hypertension or chronic kidney disease (eGFR of <60 mL/min/1.73m^2) to renal artery revascularization or medical therapy and found no benefit with revascularization.[4]

- National Kidney Foundation guidelines from 2004 state that there is insufficient evidence to recommend for or against revascularization procedures in patients with renal artery stenosis, and they recommend a case-by-case evaluation with a kidney disease specialist.[5] However, as increasing evidence mounts that revascularization is ineffective in most patients, these guidelines may require modification.[6]

Summary and Implications: The ASTRAL trial, as well as other randomized trials, demonstrate that for most patients with renal artery stenosis medical therapy is as effective as revascularization. Guidelines from the National Kidney Foundation recommend that the decision about whether to treat patients with renovascular disease with revascularization versus medical therapy should be made on a case-by-case basis. However, present data indicate that medical therapy is at least as effective as revascularization for most patients. Further research will be needed to determine which subgroups of patients, if any, benefit from revascularization.

CLINICAL CASE: MANAGEMENT OF RENAL ARTERY STENOSIS

Case History:

A 65-year-old man with a past medical history of prehypertension, diabetes, and stable angina and a 35 pack-year smoking history is found to have a blood pressure of 155/95 on physical examination and a serum creatinine of 1.8 mg/dL. Typically, his blood pressure is 130/80 and his creatinine is 1.0 mg/dL. The patient's physician initiates him on amlodipine and when he returns one month later he is found to have a blood pressure of 162/98 and a serum creatinine of 2.1 mg/dL. Renal artery imaging is ordered. The patient is found to have right-sided renal artery stenosis >70%.

Based on the results of the ASTRAL trial, how should this patient be managed?

Suggested Answer:
This patient has renal artery stenosis complicated by hypertension and kidney disease. The ASTRAL trial and other randomized trials do not suggest that patients with these conditions are likely to benefit from revascularization. Thus, it would be appropriate to treat him medically with statins, antiplatelet agents, and antihypertensives. Further research will be needed to determine whether subgroups of patients with severe disease might benefit from revascularization.

References

1. ASTRAL Investigators et al. Revascularization versus medical therapy for renal-artery stenosis. *N Engl J Med.* 2009;361:1953.
2. Kalra PA et al. The benefit of renal artery stenting in patients with atheromatous renovascular disease and advanced chronic kidney disease. *Catheter Cardiovasc Interv.* 2010;75:1.
3. Gray BH et al. Clinical benefit of renal artery angioplasty with stenting for the control of recurrent and refractory congestive heart failure. *Vasc Med.* 2002;7:275.
4. Cooper CJ et al. Stenting and medical therapy for atherosclerotic renal-artery stenosis. *N Engl J Med.* 2013;370(1):13–22.
5. Kidney Disease Outcomes Quality Initiative (K/DOQI). K/DOQI clinical practice guidelines on hypertension and antihypertensive agents in chronic kidney disease. *Am J Kidney Dis.* 2004;43:S1–S290.
6. Bitti JA. Treatment of atherosclerotic renovascular disease. *N Engl J Med.* 2014; 370:78–79.

18

Correcting Anemia in Chronic Kidney Disease

The CHOIR Trial

THOMAS KRILEY

The use of [epoetin alfa to] target a hemoglobin level of 13.5 g/dL (as compared with 11.3 g/dL) [among patients with chronic kidney disease] was associated with increased risk and no incremental improvement in the quality of life.

—SINGH ET AL.[1]

Research Question: For patients with anemia due to chronic kidney disease treated with epoetin alfa, does an aggressive hemoglobin target of 13.5 g/dL lead to better outcomes than a more conservative target of 11.3 g/dL?[1]

Funding: Johnson & Johnson Pharmaceuticals, the maker of Procrit (epoetin alfa).

Year Study Began: 2002

Year Study Published: 2006

Study Location: 130 sites in the United States.

Who Was Studied: Adults with anemia due to chronic kidney disease. To be eligible, patients were required to have a hemoglobin <11 g/dL and an estimated glomerular filtration rate (eGFR) of 15–50 mL/min/1.73m² calculated using the Modification of Diet in Renal Disease (MDRD) formula.

Who Was Excluded: Patients on renal replacement therapy at the time of enrollment. Also excluded were patients with "uncontrolled hypertension, active gastrointestinal bleeding, an iron overloaded state, a history of frequent transfusions in the last 6 months, refractory iron deficiency anemia, active cancer, previous therapy with epoetin alfa, or patients with unstable angina."[1]

How Many Patients: 1,432

Study Overview: See Figure 18.1 for a summary of the study's design.

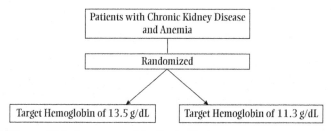

Figure 18.1 Summary of the Study Design.

Study Intervention: Patients in both groups received weekly subcutaneous injections of epoetin alfa initially at a dose of 10,000 units. After the third weekly injection, the epoetin alfa dose was adjusted to target a hemoglobin level of either 13.5 g/dL or 11.3 g/dL. The maximum dose of epoetin alfa could not exceed 20,000 units in either group, and dosing could be switched to every other week for patients with stable hemoglobin levels. Importantly, patients in both groups who began renal replacement therapy were no longer eligible to participate in the study and began receiving usual care once this occurred.

Follow-Up: Mean of 16 months.

Endpoints: Primary outcome: A composite of death, myocardial infarction, hospitalization for congestive heart failure (CHF), and stroke. Secondary outcomes: Time to renal replacement therapy; hospitalization for any cause; and changes in quality-of-life scores.

RESULTS

- Baseline characteristics in both groups were similar, with an average age of 66 years and an average baseline hemoglobin of 10.1 g/dL.
- The mean dose of epoetin alfa used and mean increase in hemoglobin level were greater in the group targeting a higher hemoglobin level (Table 18.1).
- The composite of death, myocardial infarction, hospitalization for CHF, and stroke occurred more frequently in the high hemoglobin group (Table 18.1).
- There was no statistically significant difference between groups in the need for renal replacement therapy.
- In a post hoc analysis of the primary outcome combined with the need for renal replacement therapy, there continued to be more adverse outcomes in the group targeting a higher hemoglobin.
- Changes in quality-of-life scores were similar for both groups.

Table 18.1 SUMMARY OF KEY FINDINGS

Variable	High Hemoglobin Group	Low Hemoglobin Group	P Value
Mean Change in Hemoglobin	+2.5 g/dL	+1.3 g/dL	<0.001
Mean Weekly Dose of Epoetin alfa	11,215 units	6,276 units	not reported
Primary Outcome[a]	17.5%	13.5%	0.03
Death[b]	7.3%	5.0%	0.07
Hospitalization for CHF[b]	9.0%	6.6%	0.07
Myocardial Infarction[b]	2.5%	2.8%	0.78
Stroke[b]	1.7%	1.7%	0.98

[a] Patients were only counted once for occurrence of the composite primary outcome (e.g., if hospitalization for CHF occurred before a stroke, this was counted as only one event; hospitalization for CHF was counted in the primary outcome analysis).
[b] Patients were counted for each event experienced (e.g., a patient hospitalized for CHF with subsequent stoke was counted once in each category).

Criticisms and Limitations: Of the study population, 38% did not complete follow-up (21% for unlisted reasons and 17% due to the initiation of dialysis). Because the study was unblinded, it is possible that physicians' knowledge of patients' study assignment impacted their decision to initiate dialysis, which could have biased the results. Reassuringly, however, the proportion of patients who initiated dialysis was similar between the groups, and an analysis in which dialysis initiation was combined with the primary composite outcome showed results congruent with the primary analysis.

Other Relevant Studies and Information:

- The Normal Hematocrit Trial evaluated 1,233 patients with cardiovascular disease who were on hemodialysis and found that targeting a hematocrit of 42% compared to 30% yielded no cardiovascular or mortality advantage and was associated with increased risk of thrombosis of grafts and fistulas.[2]
- In studies done after the CHOIR study of patients with chronic kidney disease and anemia who were not yet on dialysis, similar results to CHOIR's were observed; some of these studies also demonstrate an increased risk of stroke and thrombosis when targeting a higher hemoglobin level.[3,4] These trials achieved mean hemoglobin levels of 11.5 g/dL and 10.5 g/dL in the less aggressive group.
- A meta-analysis of 27 trials and 10,452 patients comparing high hemoglobin targets versus low hemoglobin targets or placebo found statistically significant increases in stoke, hypertension, and vascular thrombosis in the high hemoglobin target groups and nonstatistically significant increases in mortality and cardiovascular morbidity.[5]
- The 2012 Kidney Disease Improving Global Outcomes guidelines recommend considering initiation of erythrocyte-stimulating agents (ESAs) in patients with anemia due to chronic kidney disease who are not receiving dialysis only when hemoglobin levels fall below 10 g/dL. The decision to start treatment should be based on the rate of fall in hemoglobin and a discussion of risks and benefits with the patient. When using ESAs, the target hemoglobin should be less than 11.5 g/dL for most patients.[6] Guidelines for patients on hemodialysis recommend similar hemoglobin targets.

Summary and Implications: In patients with anemia and chronic kidney disease who are not on dialysis, using ESAs to target a hemoglobin of 13.5 g/dL is associated with increased risk compared to a target hemoglobin of 11.3 g/dL. Based on this and other research, practice guidelines recommend initiating ESAs only when the hemoglobin drops below 10 g/dL with a target hemoglobin <11.5 g/dL in most patients.

CLINICAL CASE: ANEMIA AND EPOETIN THERAPY

Case History:

A 67-year-old man with a history of hypertension, hyperlipidemia, and chronic kidney disease presents with complaints of malaise and fatigue. The patient is found to have a hemoglobin level of 10.6 g/dL with a mean cell volume (MCV) of 77 and an estimated GFR of 44 using the MDRD formula. Iron studies are ordered, which show decreased ferritin, decreased serum iron, and increased transferrin. Based on the results on the CHOIR trial, how should this patient's anemia be treated?

Suggested Answer:

Anemia associated with chronic kidney disease is typically normocytic and normochromic and related to decreased production of erythropoietin by the kidneys. The patient in this vignette, however, has microcytic anemia with iron studies suggesting iron deficiency. Prior to considering an ESA, this patient should be evaluated for iron loss and his iron stores should be repleted. If his anemia persists after treatment of his iron deficiency, an ESA still would not be recommended according to current guidelines because his hemoglobin is not <10 g/dL.

References

1. Singh AK et al. Correction of anemia with epoetin alfa in chronic kidney disease. *N Engl J Med*. 2006 Nov 16;355(20):2085–2098.
2. Besarab A et al. The effects of normal as compared with low hematocrit values in patients with cardiac disease who are receiving hemodialysis and epoetin. *N Engl J Med*. 1998;339:584.
3. Drüeke TB et al. Normalization of hemoglobin level in patients with chronic kidney disease and anemia. *N Engl J Med*. 2006;355:2071.
4. Pfeffer MA et al. A trial of darbepoetin alfa in type 2 diabetes and chronic kidney disease. *N Engl J Med*. 2009;361:2019.
5. Palmer SC et al. Meta-analysis: erythropoiesis-stimulating agents in patients with chronic kidney disease. *Ann Intern Med*. 2010;153:23.
6. Kidney Disease: Improving Global Outcomes (KDIGO) Anemia Work Group. KDIGO clinical practice guidelines for anemia in chronic kidney disease. *Kidney Int Suppl*. 2012;2:288.

19

Early versus Late Initiation of Dialysis

The IDEAL Study

MICHAEL E. HOCHMAN

> [With] careful clinical management of chronic kidney disease, dialysis
> can be delayed for some patients until the [glomerular filtration rate]
> drops below 7.0 mL per minute or until more traditional clinical indica-
> tors for the initiation of dialysis are present.
>
> —COOPER ET AL.[1]

Research Question: Can the initiation of dialysis safely be delayed in patients
with an estimated glomerular filtration rate (GFR) ≤ 14.0 mL per minute who
do not demonstrate traditional signs or symptoms indicating the need for
dialysis?[1]

Funding: Grants from several public research agencies in Australia and New
Zealand, three pharmaceutical and/or medical device companies, and by the
nonprofit International Society for Peritoneal Dialysis.

Year Study Began: 2000

Year Study Published: 2010

Study Location: 32 centers in Australia and New Zealand.

Who Was Studied: Patients ≥18 years of age with progressive chronic kidney disease and an estimated GFR between 10.0–15.0 mL per minute per 1.73 m² of body-surface area (determined using the Cockcroft-Gault equation[2] and corrected for body-surface area). Patients with kidney transplants were included in the study.

Who Was Excluded: Patients with a GFR <10.0 mL per minute, those with plans to receive a live-donor kidney transplant within the next 12 months, and those with a recently diagnosed cancer likely to impact survival.

How Many Patients: 828

Study Overview: See Figure 19.1 for a summary of the study's design.

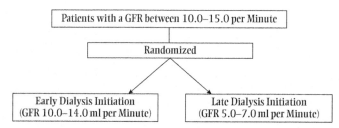

Figure 19.1 Summary of the Study Design.

Study Intervention: Patients assigned to the early dialysis group began dialysis when their GFR was between 10.0 and 14.0 mL per minute, while those assigned to the late dialysis group began dialysis when their GFR was between 5.0 and 7.0 mL per minute. Patients in the late start group could also initiate dialysis when their GFR was >7.0 mL per minute at their physicians' discretion (e.g., due to symptoms of uremia or difficult-to-manage electrolyte disturbances).

Patients and their physicians selected the method of dialysis (i.e., peritoneal dialysis versus hemodialysis) and the dialysis regimen in both groups.

Follow-Up: A median of 3.59 years.

Endpoints: Primary outcome: All-cause mortality. Secondary outcomes: Cardiovascular events (e.g., myocardial infarctions, strokes, or hospitalizations for angina); infectious events (deaths or hospitalizations due to an infection); complications of dialysis (e.g., temporary placement of an access catheter or fluid or electrolyte disorders); and quality of life.

RESULTS

- The mean age of study patients was approximately 60 years.
- The most common cause of renal failure among study patients was diabetes (approximately 34%).
- 98% of patients who survived until the end of the trial ultimately required dialysis.
- The median time until dialysis initiation in the early start group was 1.80 months versus 7.40 months in the late start group ($P < 0.001$), and the mean estimated GFR at dialysis initiation was 12.0 mL per minute in the early start group versus 9.8 mL per minute in the late start group ($P < 0.001$).
- 75.9% of patients in the late start group initiated dialysis before their GFR dropped below 7.0 due to signs or symptoms indicating the need for dialysis.
- Mortality rates were similar in patients in the early and late dialysis groups (see Table 19.1).
- Quality-of-life scores (as measured by the Assessment of Quality of Life instrument[3]) were similar between the early and late start groups.

Table 19.1 SUMMARY OF KEY FINDINGS[a]

Outcome	Early Dialysis Group	Late Dialysis Group	P Value
Death from Any Cause	10.2	9.8	0.75
Cardiovascular Events	10.9	8.8	0.09
Infectious Events	12.4	14.3	0.20
Complications of Dialysis			
Temporary Catheter Placement	10.0	9.7	0.85
Access-Site Infection	3.4	3.5	0.97
Fluid or Electrolyte Disorder	13.2	15.0	0.26

[a] Event rates are per 100 patient-years, that is, the number of events that occurred for every 100 years of patient time. For example, 10.2 deaths per 100 patient-years means that, on average, 10.2 patients died for every 25 patients who were each enrolled in the trial for 4 years.

Criticisms and Limitations: Although early dialysis initiation provided no apparent benefit, most patients in the late initiation group required dialysis during the study period before reaching a GFR of 5.0–7.0 mL per minute.

Other Relevant Studies and Information:

- An economic analysis of data from IDEAL demonstrated that dialysis costs were significantly higher in the early initiation group and total costs were nonsignificantly higher.[4]
- Other studies have suggested possible harm from dialysis initiation among patients with GFR >15.[5]
- The Kidney Disease: Improving Global Outcomes 2012 Clinical Practice Guideline for the evaluation and management of chronic kidney disease, published after the results of IDEAL were available, recommends dialysis initiation due to signs or symptoms of kidney failure, rather than at a specific GFR threshold.[6]
- Among patients who initiated dialysis in the United States in 2005, 45% had an estimated GFR >10.0 mL per minute—more than double the rate in 1996.[7]

Summary and Implications: With appropriate clinical management, patients with progressive chronic kidney disease can safely delay dialysis initiation until they either develop signs or symptoms indicating the need for dialysis or until their GFR drops below 7.0 mL per minute. Although most patients in the late start group required dialysis before their GFR dropped below 7.0, patients were able to delay dialysis initiation by an average of 6 months without any adverse effects.

CLINICAL CASE: EARLY VERSUS LATE INITIATION OF DIALYSIS

Case History:

A 56-year-old woman with chronic kidney disease due to diabetes presents for an initial evaluation in the nephrology clinic at an urban medical center. The patient was referred for nephrology consultation almost 2 years ago. However, there is a long backlog for nephrology appointments, and the nephrologists are overwhelmed with patients. The woman is currently asymptomatic, and her estimated GFR is 12 mL per minute. Her physical examination is normal, as are her electrolytes.

As a nephrologist in this clinic, and based on the results of the IDEAL trial, do you feel comfortable delaying dialysis initiation in this patient until she develops a "hard" indication such as a difficult-to-manage electrolyte disturbance?

Suggested Answer:

The IDEAL trial demonstrated that, with appropriate monitoring, patients with progressive chronic kidney disease can safely delay dialysis initiation until they either develop signs or symptoms indicating the need for dialysis or until their GFR drops below 7.0 mL per minute. Thus, under ideal circumstances, the patient in this vignette would be able to delay dialysis initiation.

This patient receives care at an underresourced medical center, however, and the nephrology staff may not be able to monitor her closely over the next several months. Without appropriate monitoring, this patient is at risk for a life-threatening complication. Thus, given the resource limitations, it might be appropriate to initiate dialysis immediately.

References

1. Cooper BA et al. A randomized, controlled trial of early vs. late initiation of dialysis. *N Engl J Med.* 2010 Aug 12;363(7):609–619.
2. Cockcroft DW, Gault MH. Prediction of creatinine clearance from serum creatinine. *Nephron.* 1976;16:31–41.
3. Hawthorne G et al. The Assessment of Quality of Life (AQoL) instrument: a psychometric measure of health-related quality of life. *Qual Life Res.* 1999;8:209–224.
4. Harris A et al. Cost-effectiveness of initiating dialysis early: a randomized controlled trial. *Am J Kidney Dis.* 2011;57(5):707–715.
5. Susantitaphong P et al. GFR at initiation of dialysis and mortality in CKD: a meta-analysis. *Am J Kidney Dis.* 2012;59(6):829.
6. Kidney Disease: Improving Global Outcomes CKD Work Group. KDIGO 2012 Clinical Practice Guideline for the Evaluation and Management of Chronic Kidney Disease. *Kidney Int Suppl.* 2013;3:5.
7. Rosansky SJ et al. Initiation of dialysis at higher GFRs: is the apparent rising tide of early dialysis harmful or helpful? *Kidney Int.* 2009;76:257–261.

Gastroenterology

20

Use of IV Albumin in Patients with Cirrhosis and Spontaneous Bacterial Peritonitis

STEVEN D. HOCHMAN

> We found that the administration of albumin prevents renal impairment and reduces mortality in patients with cirrhosis and spontaneous bacterial peritonitis.
>
> —SORT ET AL.[1]

Research Question: Does the administration of IV albumin improve survival in patients admitted to the hospital with cirrhosis and spontaneous bacterial peritonitis?[1]

Funding: Grants from the Spanish Health Research Fund and the Hospital Clinic, an autonomous scientific and technical body associated with the national organization tasked with funding public health in Spain.

Year Study Began: 1995

Year Study Published: 1999

Study Location: Seven university hospitals in Spain.

Who Was Studied: Patients 18 to 80 years of age with cirrhosis admitted to the hospital with spontaneous bacterial peritonitis (SBP), defined by an ascitic fluid polymorphonuclear cell count of >250 per cubic millimeter.

Who Was Excluded: Patients with "findings suggestive of secondary peritonitis." In addition, patients with recent use of antibiotics other than prophylactic norfloxacin, current infections other than SBP, "shock, gastrointestinal bleeding, ileus, grade 3 or 4 hepatic encephalopathy, cardiac failure, organic nephropathy, or other diseases that could affect short term mortality."[1] Those with creatinine >3 mg/dL or other causes of dehydration were also excluded.

How Many Patients: 126

Study Overview: See Figure 20.1 for a summary of the study's design.

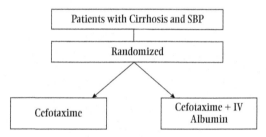

Figure 20.1 Summary of the Study Design.

Study Intervention: All patients were administered intravenous cefotaxime, renally dosed based on the admission creatinine level. Patients in the albumin plus cefotaxime group also received a 1.5 grams per kilogram of body-weight dose of intravenous albumin within 6 hours of enrollment, and a 1 gram per kilogram of body-weight dose of intravenous albumin on day 3 after enrollment. Diuretic treatment and therapeutic paracentesis were not allowed in either group until the infection had resolved. However, a small number of patients in both groups received a partial paracentesis, with aspiration of 3 liters, before resolution of the infection.

Follow-Up: 90 days.

Endpoints: (1) Resolution of infection, defined by disappearance of signs of infection and an ascitic fluid polymorphonuclear cell count less than 250 per cubic millimeter. (2) Renal failure, defined as nonreversible deterioration of renal function during hospitalization. For patients with renal disease at the time on enrollment (blood urea nitrogen [BUN] ≥30 mg/dL or Cr ≥1.5 mg/dL on admission), this was defined as a rise in BUN or creatinine of more than 50% from baseline. For patients without renal disease at the time of enrollment, this was defined as a rise in BUN or creatinine of more than 50% from baseline if the rise resulted in a BUN >30 mg/dL or creatinine >1.5 mg/dL. (3) Mortality while in the hospital and 3 months after enrollment.

RESULTS

- Though resolution of infections occurred with equal frequency in both groups, patients treated with intravenous albumin experienced less renal impairment and lower mortality than those receiving cefotaxime alone (Table 20.1).
- The benefits of IV albumin were most pronounced among patients with a baseline bilirubin ≥4 mg/dL or baseline creatinine ≥1 mg/dL.
- Patients treated with cefotaxime alone were more likely to have high plasma renin activity, and patients with an increase in renin activity were more likely to develop renal impairment, suggesting that albumin administration benefited patients by improving intravascular volume and renal perfusion.

Table 20.1 SUMMARY OF KEY FINDINGS

	Cefotaxime	Cefotaxime + Albumin	P Value
Resolution of Infection	94%	98%	0.36
Renal Impairment	33%	10%	0.002
In-Hospital Mortality	29%	10%	0.01
Mortality at 3 Months	41%	22%	0.03

Criticisms and Limitations: The study has been criticized for not describing the fluid management of patients during their hospitalization.

Other Relevant Studies and Information:

- A 2007 trial of 28 patients with 38 cases of SBP was consistent with the results of this trial among high-risk patients. However, it found that patients with low-risk SBP (bilirubin <4 mg/dL, Cr <1 mg/dL, and BUN <30 mg/dL) did not benefit from the administration of IV albumin.[2]

- A meta-analysis of 4 studies involving 288 patients found a reduction in renal impairment (8% versus 31%) and mortality (16% versus 35%) when using IV albumin to treat SBP.[3]
- Guidelines from the American Association for the Study of Liver Diseases recommend the use of IV albumin among patients with SBP and a total bilirubin >4 mg/dL, creatinine >1 mg/dL, *or* BUN >30 mg/dL.[4]

Summary and Implications: This was the first randomized trial to establish the effectiveness of IV albumin for the treatment of SBP among high-risk patients with cirrhosis. Guidelines now recommend IV albumin for patients with SBP who have an elevated total bilirubin, serum creatinine, or blood urea nitrogen.

CLINICAL CASE: CIRRHOTIC PATIENT WITH ABDOMINAL DISTENTION

Case History:

A 59-year-old man with a history of alcoholic cirrhosis presents with 4 days of increasing abdominal girth, abdominal pain, and subjective fevers. On physical examination, he has a temperature of 101.1°F, and the abdomen is distended, with shifting dullness, and is diffusely tender to palpation without rebound or guarding. Diagnostic paracentesis performed prior to antibiotic administration shows 4,747 polymorphonuclear cells per cubic millimeter. Ascitic fluid culture is pending. A basic metabolic panel drawn on admission shows sodium, 135; potassium, 4.4; chloride, 101; bicarbonate, 23; BUN, 22; creatinine, 1.2; and glucose, 132. The total serum bilirubin is 3.2 mg/dL.

Based on the results of this trial, how should this patient be treated?

Suggested Answer:

This patient, who has increasing abdominal girth, fevers, and abdominal tenderness, most likely has spontaneous bacterial peritonitis, which was confirmed by diagnostic paracentesis demonstrating >250 polymorphonuclear cells per cubic millimeter of ascitic fluid. Though cultures of ascitic fluid are still pending, this patient should be immediately started on a third-generation cephalosporin, with refinement of the antibiotics based on culture results and susceptibility testing. This patient has a baseline creatinine of 1.2 and is at high risk for the development of renal impairment. Thus he should also be started on IV albumin with an infusion of 1.5 g/kg given now and 1 g/kg given 3 days later.

References

1. Sort P et al. Effects of intravenous albumin on renal impairment and mortality in patients with cirrhosis and spontaneous bacterial peritonitis. *N Engl J Med.* 1999;341:403.
2. Sigal S, Stanca C, Fernandez J, Arroyo V, Navasa M. Restricted use of albumin for spontaneous bacterial peritonitis. *Gut* 2007;56:597.
3. Salerno F, Navickis RJ, Wilkes MM. Albumin infusion improves outcomes of patients with spontaneous bacterial peritonitis: a meta analysis of randomized trials. *Clin Gastroenterol Hepatol.* 2013;11:123.
4. Runyon B, AASLD Practice Guidelines Committee. Management of adult patients with ascites due to cirrhosis: an update. *Hepatology* 2009;49(6):2087.

21

Early Use of Transjugular Intrahepatic Portosystemic Shunt (TIPS) in Patients with Cirrhosis and Variceal Bleeding

ADEL BOUEIZ

In these patients with cirrhosis who were hospitalized for acute variceal bleeding and at high risk for treatment failure, the early use of TIPS was associated with significant reductions in treatment failure and in mortality . . . [However], because of [previous] findings, TIPS is [still] currently recommended only as a rescue therapy.

—GARCÍA-PAGÁN ET AL.[1]

Research Question: For high-risk patients with cirrhosis and acute variceal bleeding, is early treatment with transjugular intrahepatic portosystemic shunts (TIPS) better than drug therapy plus endoscopic band ligation?[1]

Funding: W. L. Gore and Associates, the maker of the extended polytetrafluoroethylene (e-PTFE)-covered stents used in the study, as well as several government and academic institutions in Spain and France.

Year Study Began: 2004

Year Study Published: 2010

Study Location: Nine centers in Europe.

Who Was Studied: Adults with Child-Pugh class B or C cirrhosis admitted in the previous 12 hours with acute variceal bleeding who were being treated with endoscopic therapy, prophylactic antibiotics, and vasoactive medications. To be eligible for inclusion, patients were required to have either Child-Pugh class C cirrhosis (a score of 10 to 13) or class B cirrhosis (a score of 7 to 9) accompanied by "active bleeding at diagnostic endoscopy."

Who Was Excluded: Patients with severe cirrhosis (Child-Pugh score >13) were excluded as were patients with previous treatment with combined pharmacologic and endoscopic therapy or TIPS to prevent variceal rebleeding. In addition, patients were excluded if they were >75 years old, had hepatocellular carcinoma not amenable to transplantation, had a serum creatinine >3 mg/dL, or had "bleeding from isolated gastric or ectopic varices."

How Many Patients: 63

Study Overview: See Figure 21.1 for a summary of the study design.

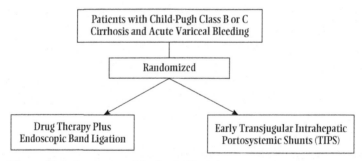

Figure 21.1 Summary of the Study Design.

Study Intervention: All patients in both groups were treated initially with vasoactive medications, prophylactic antibiotics, and endoscopic therapy (band ligation or sclerotherapy).

Patients randomized to drug therapy plus endoscopic band ligation were managed with vasoactive drugs until they were "free of bleeding for a minimum of 24 hours" and ideally for up to 5 days, at which point they were transitioned to therapy with nonselective beta blockers and isosorbide-5-mononitrate. Patients in this group also received elective endoscopic band ligation at 7–14 days following initial endoscopic treatment and then "every 10–14 days thereafter until variceal eradication was achieved." Surveillance endoscopy was performed 1, 6, and 12 months after eradication with endoscopic band ligation for recurrent varices. Patients who experienced a single rebleeding episode requiring transfusion with two or more units of blood or multiple less-severe rebleeding episodes were eligible for TIPS as "rescue therapy."

Patients randomized to early TIPS received TIPS with placement of an e-PTFE-covered stent within 72 hours of the initial diagnostic endoscopy. The stent was initially dilated to 8 mm but if the portal pressure gradient (pressure difference between the portal vein and inferior vena cava) did not fall to <12 mm Hg, the stent was dilated to 10 mm. TIPS revision with angioplasty or stent replacement was performed if there was "clinical recurrence of portal hypertension or evidence of TIPS dysfunction on ultrasound."

Follow-Up: Median follow-up was 10.6 months in the endoscopic therapy group and 14.6 months in the TIPS group.

Endpoints: Primary outcome: A composite of bleeding episodes ("failure to control acute bleeding or failure to prevent recurrent clinically significant variceal rebleeding within 1 year"). Secondary outcomes: Mortality and time spent in the intensive care unit or hospital.

RESULTS

- Of 359 patients admitted for acute variceal bleeding during the enrollment period, only 63 underwent randomization; many were excluded based on their Child-Pugh score (72 were class A, 40 were class B without active bleeding, and 18 had scores >13).
- Baseline characteristics were similar between the two groups with an average age of 50 years; 67% of patients were male.
- In the endoscopy therapy group, variceal eradication was achieved in 52% of patients.
- In the TIPS group, the procedure was carried out without major complications in all but one patient who withdrew consent, and in all but two patients portal-pressure gradient dropped below 12 mm Hg following the procedure.
- Early use of TIPS was associated with reduced risk of bleeding events and mortality compared with endoscopic therapy (Table 21.1).

- Of 14 patients in the endoscopic therapy group experiencing bleeding events, 7 received TIPS with e-PTFE-covered stents as "rescue therapy"; 4 of these 7 died within 36 days.
- There were no between-group differences in the occurrence of hepatic encephalopathy, ascites, spontaneous bacterial peritonitis, or hepatorenal syndrome.

Table 21.1. SUMMARY OF KEY FINDINGS

Outcome	TIPS	Endoscopic Therapy	P Value
Failure to Control Acute Bleeding or Prevent Rebleeding	3%	45%	0.001
Mortality	13%	39%	0.01
Hepatic Encephalopathy	25%	39%	nonsignificant
Percentage of Follow-Up in the Hospital	4%	15%	0.014
Days in the ICU	3.6	8.6	0.01

Criticisms and Limitations: Only a small percentage of very high risk patients admitted with acute variceal bleeding were eligible for the trial. Thus these results only apply to a small subset of very high risk patients (i.e. those with Child-Pugh class C cirrhosis or class B cirrhosis with active bleeding).

Other Relevant Studies:

- A meta-analysis of 11 trials and 801 patients concluded that, for patients with acute variceal bleeding, TIPS was associated with a reduced rate of rebleeding, an increased rate of hepatic encephalopathy, and no difference in mortality compared to endoscopic therapy.[2] However, most prior studies used bare stents (rather than the e-PTFE-covered stents used in this trial), and many trials excluded high-risk patients who were included in this study.
- Guidelines from the American Association for the Study of Liver Disease recommend TIPS only as salvage therapy in patients with uncontrolled variceal bleeding that does not respond to endoscopic therapy.[3] These guidelines were issued prior to the publication of this trial, however.

Summary and Implications: This study demonstrates the benefits of TIPS among a subset of very high-risk patients with acute variceal bleeding and Child-Pugh class B or C cirrhosis. Unlike prior studies that focused on a broad population of patients with variceal bleeding, this study was limited to a very high-risk group (those with Child-Pugh class C cirrhosis or class B cirrhosis with active bleeding). Based on prior research, current guidelines still recommend TIPS only as salvage therapy for variceal bleeding not responsive to endoscopic therapy. However, this study suggests a benefit of early TIPS among a subset of high-risk patients and underscores the need for more research.

CLINICAL CASE: MANAGEMENT OF ACUTE VARICEAL BLEEDING

Case History:

A 68-year-old man hospitalized for advanced cirrhosis complicated by ascites and encephalopathy is evaluated for massive hematemesis and hypotension. The patient's medications are spironolactone, furosemide, and lactulose. His stool is black and positive for blood. Laboratory studies show hemoglobin of 9 g/dL, a platelet count of 60,000/μL, and an international normalized ratio (INR) of 2.2. His calculated Child-Pugh score is 13. Upper endoscopy reveals actively bleeding esophageal varices.

In addition to rapid volume resuscitation and antibiotics, what treatment would you recommend for this patient?

Suggested Answer:

This study found that early TIPS reduced bleeding episodes and mortality among high-risk patients like the one in this vignette with active variceal bleeding. Although current guidelines recommend TIPS only as a salvage therapy, it would be reasonable to consider early TIPS in this patient because he is similar to the high-risk patients included in this study. On the other hand, because this patient suffers from hepatic encephalopathy, an initial endoscopic approach would also be reasonable because TIPS has been implicated as a cause of worsening encephalopathy in prior research.

References

1. García-Pagán JC et al. Early use of TIPS in patients with cirrhosis and variceal bleeding. *N Engl J Med.* 2010 June 24;362(25):2370–2379.
2. Papatheodoridis GV et al. Transjugular intrahepatic portosystemic shunt compared with endoscopic treatment for prevention of variceal rebleeding: a meta-analysis. *Hepatology* 1999;30:612.
3. Garcia-Tsao G et al. Prevention and management of gastroesophageal varices and variceal hemorrhage in cirrhosis. *Hepatology* 2007;46(3):922–938.

Infectious Diseases

22

Methicillin-Resistant *S. aureus* Infections among Patients in the Emergency Department

LAALITHA SURAPANENI

> MRSA is now the most common pathogen isolated in the emergency department from patients with [purulent] skin and soft-tissue infections with an average prevalence of 59%.
>
> —MORAN ET AL.[1]

Research Question: Among adults with purulent skin and soft tissue infections presenting to emergency departments (EDs), what is the prevalence and antibiotic susceptibility of methicillin-resistant *Staphylococcus aureus* (MRSA)?[1]

Funding: Centers for Disease Control and Prevention.

Year Study Began: 2004

Year Study Published: 2006

Study Location: 11 university-affiliated EDs in the United States.

Who Was Studied: Adult patients with purulent skin or soft tissue infections.

Who Was Excluded: Patients with infections present for more than 1 week and those with perirectal abscesses.

How Many Patients: 422

Study Overview: See Figure 22.1 for an overview of the study's design.

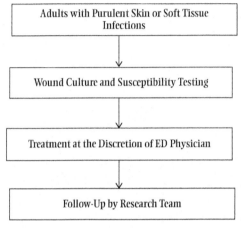

Figure 22.1 Summary of the Study Design.

Study Intervention: For patients presenting with purulent skin or soft tissue infections, the "single largest area of infection" was sampled for culture and antibiotic susceptibility testing at the local hospital's laboratory. A subset of samples was forwarded to the laboratories at the Centers for Disease Control and Prevention for further analysis of bacterial genetics and antibiotic susceptibility testing. Patients were treated at the discretion of the local ED physician. Research staff followed up with patients by telephone 2 to 3 weeks after their initial presentation.

Follow-Up: 2–3 weeks.

Outcomes: Prevalence of MRSA; MRSA susceptibility patterns; and risk factors associated with MRSA infection.

RESULTS:

- The median age of patients was 39 years; 62% were male. Approximately half were black; one-quarter were white; and one quarter were Hispanic.
- 81% of the presenting infections were abscesses, 11% were infected wounds, and 8% were cellulitis with purulent exudate.
- MRSA was the most common bacterial species isolated from infections overall, followed by methicillin-sensitive *S. aureus* (MSSA) and *Streptococcus* species (Table 22.1).
- MRSA was the most commonly isolated bacterial species at 10 of the 11 EDs.
- 99% of MRSA isolates were characterized as community-acquired based on genetic data.
- 100% of the MRSA isolates were susceptible to trimethoprim-sulfamethoxazole and rifampin; 95% were susceptible to clindamycin; 92% to tetracycline; 60% to fluoroquinolones; and 6% to erythromycin.
- Several features were identified as factors affecting the risk for MRSA infection (Table 22.2); however, 31% of patients who experienced a MRSA infection had none of the identified risk factors.
- Of all patients, 19% were treated with incision and drainage alone, 10% with antibiotics alone, 66% with both, and 5% with neither; in 57% of patients with MRSA, antibiotic treatment was not concordant with susceptibility testing.
- 59% of patients were contacted 2–3 weeks following initial presentation, of whom 96% reported that their infection was resolved or improved; there were no differences in response between those with MRSA versus other isolates or those with MRSA isolates that were susceptible versus resistant to the prescribed antibiotic.

Table 22.1 Bacteria Isolated from Infection Cultures

Bacteria	Percentage of Infected Wounds
Methicillin-Resistant *S. aureus*	59%
Methicillin-Sensitive *S. aureus*	17%
Streptococcus species	7%
Other	8%
No Bacterial Growth	9%

Table 22.2 FEATURES ASSOCIATED WITH MRSA INFECTION

Variable	Odds Ratio (95% Confidence Interval)
Use of Antibiotics in the Last Month	2.4 (1.4–4.1)
Presence of an Abscess	1.8 (1.0–3.1)
Reported Spider Bite	2.8 (1.5–4.3)
History of MRSA Infection	3.3 (1.2–10.1)
Contact with Person with Similar Infection	3.4 (1.5–8.1)
Race Other Than Black, White, or Hispanic	0.3 (0.1–0.9)
Underlying Illness	0.3 (0.2–0.6)

Criticisms and Limitations: Variability of the results between centers may make it difficult to generalize these findings to all clinical settings. Additionally, antibiotic resistance patterns evolve over time due to selection pressures and thus this analysis will need to be repeated frequently to ensure the results continue to be clinically relevant.

Other Relevant Studies and Information:

- The same research group performed a similar study in 2008 and found a similar prevalence of MRSA infections and bacterial susceptibilities, but with less variation among sites. In the 2008 study, a higher proportion of patients were treated empirically for MRSA infections.[2]
- A study of 384 individuals with purulent skin infections caused by *S. aureus* found that 72% of infections were caused by MRSA, of which 87% were strains of community-acquired MRSA.[3]
- The Infectious Diseases Society of America practice guidelines recommend incision and drainage as the primary treatment for cutaneous abscesses, with addition of empiric antibiotics with MRSA coverage (e.g., trimethoprim-sulfamethoxazole or clindamycin) for severe infections such as those >5 cm or when there is extensive surrounding cellulitis, systemic symptoms, associated comorbidities, or immunosuppression.[4]

Summary and Implications: Among patients presenting with purulent skin and soft tissue infections, MRSA was the most commonly pathogen identified at 11 EDs. Although incision and drainage are the main treatments for most patients with such infections, empiric treatment with MRSA coverage should be used when antibiotics are indicated (e.g., severe infections or when the host is immunocompromised).

CLINICAL CASE: MRSA PREVALENCE IN THE COMMUNITY

Case History:
A 24-year-old man presents to the ED with a 6-cm abscess in his axilla for the past 3 days. In addition to incision and drainage, what antibiotics should be given to this patient upon discharge?

Suggested Answer:
This study found that MRSA is the most common cause of purulent skin infections such as the abscess in this patient. Given the size of the abscess, the patient would likely benefit from antibiotic therapy in addition to incision and drainage. Until culture and susceptibility results are available, the patient should be started on empiric antibiotics with MRSA coverage, such as trimethoprim-sulfamethoxazole or clindamycin.

References

1 Moran GJ et al. Methicillin-resistant S. *aureus* infections among patients in the emergency department. *N Engl J Med.* 2006;355:666–674.
2 Talan DA et al. Comparison of Staphylococcus aureus from skin and soft tissue infections in U.S. emergency department patients, 2004 and 2008. *Clin Infect Dis.* 2011 Jul;53(2):144–149.
3 King MD, Humphrey BJ, Wany YF, Kourbatova EV, Ray SM, Blumberg HM. Emergency of community-acquired methicillin-resistant *Staphylococcus aureus* USA 300 clone as the predominant cause of skin and soft tissue infections. *Ann Intern Med.* 2006;144:309–317.
4 Liu C. Clinical Practice Guidelines by the Infectious Diseases Society of America for the treatment of methicillin-resistant *Staphylococcus aureus* infections in adults and children. *Clin Infect Dis.* 2011;52(3):q18–55.

23

Antibiotic Therapy in Exacerbations of Chronic Obstructive Pulmonary Disease

KRISTOPHER SWIGER

This study shows that, compared with placebo, antibiotic treatment of chronic obstructive pulmonary disease in exacerbation produced significantly earlier resolution of symptoms.

—ANTHONISEN ET AL.[1]

Research Question: Should patients with exacerbations of chronic obstructive pulmonary disease (COPD) be treated with antibiotics?[1]

Funding: Health and Welfare Canada, a government organization.

Year Study Began: 1981

Year Study Published: 1987

Study Location: One university center in Canada.

Who Was Studied: Patients over the age of 35 with a clinical diagnosis of COPD and a forced expiratory volume in 1 second (FEV1) ≤70% of the predicted value and a total lung capacity ≥80% of the predicted value.

Who Was Excluded: Patients were excluded if the FEV1 increased to >80% of the predicted value with the use of an inhaled bronchodilator (consistent with reversible airway disease). Patients were also excluded if they had other diseases "serious enough to influence their clinical course" (e.g., cancer, heart failure, stroke) or conditions "likely to require antibiotic therapy" (e.g., recurrent sinusitis or urinary tract infections).

How Many Patients: 173

Study Overview: See Figure 23.1 for a summary of the study's design.

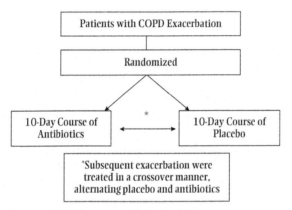

Figure 23.1 Summary of the Study Design.

Study Intervention: All patients were maintained on a standard regimen of inhaled or nebulized albuterol and oral theophylline, as well as oral prednisone and/or home oxygen as needed. Patients self-reported exacerbations by phone and were scheduled for a same-day appointment with nurse-practitioners, who assessed symptoms by a standardized questionnaire and determined if the patient was experiencing an exacerbation. Exacerbations were classified into three types as follows:

- Type 1: Increased dyspnea, sputum volume, and sputum purulence
- Type 2: Two of the above symptoms
- Type 3: One of the above symptoms in addition to one of the following: upper respiratory infection, fever, increased wheezing or coughing, or increases in respiratory rate or heart rate by 20% relative to baseline

Patients deemed to have an exacerbation of any type were randomized to receive antibiotic therapy or placebo for 10 days. Within the antibiotic treatment group, patients were randomized to receive trimethoprim-sulfamethoxazole 160 mg or 180 mg twice daily, amoxicillin 250 mg four times daily, or doxycycline 200 mg initially and then 100 mg once daily.

Follow-Up: Mean of 23.7 months ± 11.3 months.

Endpoints: "Treatment success," defined as resolution of all symptoms accompanying the exacerbation within 21 days. A subset of patients was also assessed for the functional endpoint of peak flow measurement recovery.

RESULTS

- Patients were predominantly male (80%), with a mean age of 67 years.
- The 173 patients enrolled experienced 362 exacerbations during the study period (average of one exacerbation every 9.2 months).
- Treatment success rate was higher for those receiving antibiotics compared to placebo (Table 23.1).
- Peak flow recovered more rapidly in patients treated with antibiotics compared to those treated with placebo.
- Patients with a type 1 exacerbation (i.e., patients with all three of the symptoms defining an exacerbation) benefited most from antibiotics relative to placebo.

Table 23.1 SUMMARY OF KEY FINDINGS

Outcome	Placebo	Antibiotic	P Value
Treatment Success	55.0%	68.1%	<0.01
Failure with Deterioration Requiring Additional Therapy	18.9%	9.9%	<0.05
Treatment Discontinued	2.5%	1.5%	<0.05

Criticisms and Limitations: The definition of a COPD exacerbation used in this study (the "Anthonisen definition") is considered to be narrow in scope because it does not include several important symptoms such as chest congestion, chest tightness, fatigue, and sleep disturbances. Additionally, it may not exclude similarly presenting diagnoses, such as heart failure or pneumonia.

Additionally, patients with mild COPD were poorly represented in this trial.

Other Relevant Studies and Information:

- Two systematic reviews conclude that antibiotics reduce the risk of treatment failure and improve mortality among patients with severe exacerbations requiring hospitalization.[2,3]
- A meta-analysis of mild COPD exacerbations presenting in the outpatient setting found no reduction in the risk of treatment failure with versus without antibiotic administration when restricting the analysis to studies of currently available antibiotic therapies.[3]
- The Global Initiative for Chronic Obstructive Lung Disease (GOLD) supports the use of antibiotics for moderate or severely ill patients with COPD exacerbations with sputum purulence combined with increased dyspnea and/or increased sputum volume or those requiring mechanical ventilation.[4]

Summary and Implications: This trial demonstrated the benefit of antibiotics (trimethoprim-sulfamethoxazole, amoxicillin, or doxycycline) in patients with exacerbations of COPD who have three cardinal symptoms: increased dyspnea, increased sputum volume, and increased sputum purulence. Other studies have failed to demonstrate a benefit of antibiotics among patients with milder forms of COPD. Based on these findings, guidelines support the use of antibiotics for patients with moderate or severe exacerbations of COPD who have sputum purulence combined with increased dyspnea and/or increased sputum volume or those requiring mechanical ventilation.

CLINICAL CASE: COPD EXACERBATION

Case History:
A 56-year-old man with moderate COPD presents to the emergency room with four days of escalating dyspnea, cough, and new purulent sputum production. He has been using his albuterol inhaler very frequently in the last 2 days without sustained relief. He reports that he normally coughs up some sputum every morning but notes that the volume has increased. In addition, while his sputum usually is white or clear, it now appears green. Based on the trial by Anthonisen et al., how should this patient be treated?

Suggested Answer:
This study demonstrated the benefit of antibiotics among patients with moderate to severe COPD exacerbations. Patients most likely to benefit from antibiotics include those with all three cardinal symptoms of a COPD exacerbation: increased dyspnea, sputum volume, and sputum purulence. The patient in this vignette has all three of these symptoms and thus is likely to benefit from antibiotics. Thus, in concordance with the above trial and current guidelines, this patient should be offered an antibiotic for a course of 5–10 days. The antibiotic choice should be informed by local resistance patterns.

References

1. Anthonisen NR et al. Antibiotic therapy in exacerbations of chronic obstructive pulmonary disease. *Annals Intern Med.* 1987;106:196–204.
2. Quon BS, Gan WQ, Sin DD. Contemporary management of acute exacerbations of COPD: a systematic review and meta analysis. *Chest.* 2008;133:756–766.
3. Vollenweider DJ, Jarrett H, Steurer-Stey CA et al. Antibiotics for exacerbations of chronic obstructive pulmonary disease. *Cochrane Database Syst Rev.* 2012;12:CD010257.
4. Vestbo J et al. Global strategy for the diagnosis, management, and prevention of chronic obstructive pulmonary disease: GOLD executive summary. *Amer J Resp Crit Care Med.* 2013;187(4):347–365.

Early versus Delayed Antiretroviral Therapy for Patients with HIV

The NA-ACCORD Study

MICHAEL E. HOCHMAN

The results of this study suggest that among patients with a 351–500 CD4+ count, the deferral of antiretroviral therapy was associated with an increase in the risk of death of 69% . . . Among patients with a more-than-500 CD4+ count, deferred therapy was associated with an increase in the risk of death of 94% . . . [However] since patients in our study did not undergo randomization, the decision to initiate or defer antiretroviral therapy could have been influenced by multiple factors.

—KITAHATA ET AL.[1]

Research Question: At what CD4+ count should antiretroviral therapy be initiated in asymptomatic patients with HIV?[1]

Funding: The National Institutes of Health, and the Agency for Healthcare Research and Quality.

Year Study Began: Data from 1996 to 2005 were included.

Year Study Published: 2009

Study Location: Data are from more than 60 sites in the United States and Canada.

Who Was Studied: A cohort of asymptomatic US and Canadian patients with HIV. Two separate analyses were performed: one involving patients with a CD4+ count of 351–500 cells per cubic millimeter and another in patients with a CD4+ count >500 cells per cubic millimeter.

Who Was Excluded: Patients with a previous AIDS-defining illness and those who had previously received antiretroviral therapy (ART).

How Many Patients: 17,517

Study Overview: See Figure 24.1 for a summary of the study's design.

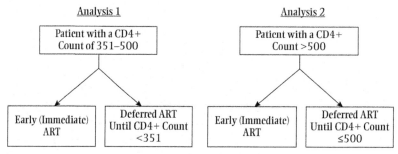

Figure 24.1 Summary of the Study Design.

- Because this was not a randomized trial, patients chose whether they would receive early versus deferred ART.
- The authors adjusted the results for differences between patients in the early versus deferred ART groups (e.g., for differences in baseline age and CD4+ count).

Study Intervention: In the first analysis, patients in the early therapy group received ART when their CD4+ counts were 351–500. Patients in the deferred therapy group did not receive ART until their counts were <351. Patients who initiated ART more than 6 months after having a measured CD4+ count of 351–500 but before their counts dropped below 351 were excluded.

In the second analysis, patients in the early therapy group received ART when their CD4+ counts were >500. Patients in the deferred therapy group did not receive ART until their counts were ≤500. Patients who initiated ART more than 6 months after having a measured CD4+ count of >500 but before their counts were ≤500 were excluded.

Follow-Up: Mean of 2.9 years.

Endpoint: Death.

RESULTS

Analysis 1: CD4+ Count 351–500

- 8,362 patients were eligible for analysis 1, and of these patients 25% initiated early ART.
- Patients in the early therapy group were more likely to be white men and less likely to have a history of intravenous drug use and hepatitis C.
- Patients in the early therapy group had a lower mortality rate than those in the deferred therapy group (see Table 24.1).

Table 24.1 SUMMARY OF KEY FINDINGS OF ANALYSIS 1

Outcome	Mortality Rate in Deferred ART Group[a]	Mortality Rate in Early ART Group[a]	Adjusted Odds Ratio for Deferred versus Early ART	P Value
Death	5%	3%	1.69	<0.001

[a] Because of the complexity of these analyses, these rates are only approximate.

Analysis 2: CD4+ >500

- 9,155 patients were eligible for analysis 2, and of these patients 24% initiated early ART.
- Patients in the early therapy group were more likely to be white men and less likely to have a history of intravenous drug use and hepatitis C.
- Patients in the early therapy group had a higher rate of viral suppression after therapy initiation than patients in the deferred therapy group (81% versus 71%), suggesting better medication compliance in the early therapy group.
- Patients in the early therapy group had a lower mortality rate than those in the deferred therapy group (see Table 24.2).

Table 24.2 SUMMARY OF KEY FINDINGS OF ANALYSIS 2

Outcome	Mortality Rate in Deferred ART Group[a]	Mortality Rate in Early ART Group[a]	Adjusted Odds Ratio for Deferred versus Early ART	P Value
Death	5.1%	2.6%	1.94	<0.001

[a] Because of the complexity of these analyses, these rates are only approximate.

Criticisms and Limitations: The major limitation of NA-ACCORD is that it was not a randomized trial and even though the authors tried to adjust for differences between patients in the early versus delayed therapy groups, it is possible that unmeasured confounding factors could have affected the results. For example, patients in the early therapy group may have been more engaged in their health than patients in the deferred therapy group, which may have led to improved survival among the early therapy patients. Indeed, patients in the early therapy group from analysis 2 had a higher rate of viral suppression than patients in the delayed ART group, suggesting a higher rate of medication compliance among early ART patients.

Another limitation of NA-ACCORD is that the authors did not report data on medication toxicity.

Other Relevant Studies and Information:

- High-quality randomized trials have convincingly demonstrated the benefit of ART in patients with a CD4+ count ≤200. In addition, strong evidence suggests that ART is beneficial in patients with CD4+ counts in the range of 200–350.[2]
- The HPTN 052 trial showed that initiation of ART in patients with a CD4+ count between 350 and 550 reduced rates of sexual HIV transmission and HIV-related complications, most notably extrapulmonary tuberculosis.[3]
- The SMART trial also suggested a benefit of ART in patients with CD4+ counts >350.[4,5]
- Based in part on data from NA-ACCORD, 2014 guidelines from the International Antiviral Society-USA Panel recommend the initiation of ART in all adults with HIV, though the guidelines acknowledge that the strength of the evidence increases "with decreasing CD4 cell count and the presence of certain concurrent conditions."[6]
- A number of randomized trials are underway to more definitively determine the optimal strategy for initiating ART in asymptomatic patients.

Summary and Implications: Although NA-ACCORD was not a randomized trial and therefore the conclusions are far from definitive, the results suggest that initiation of ART in asymptomatic patients with HIV is beneficial when the CD4+ count is 351–500 as well as when the count is >500.

CLINICAL CASE: EARLY VERSUS DELAYED ANTIRETROVIRAL THERAPY FOR PATIENTS WITH HIV

Case History:

A 34-year-old man with a history of intravenous drug use presents to your HIV clinic for a follow-up evaluation. He has missed three out of his last four clinic appointments, and he admits to continued intermittent IV drug use. His most recent CD4+ count, measured 2 months ago, was 542, and his viral load was 36,000 copies/mL. The patient asks you if he should start taking medications to treat his HIV.

Based on the results of NA-ACCORD, how should you respond?

Suggested Answer:

NA-ACCORD suggests that initiation of ART in asymptomatic patients with HIV and a CD4+ count >500 is beneficial. Based in part on these results, 2014 guidelines recommend the initiation of ART in all patients with HIV, regardless of the CD4+ count. Still, NA-ACCORD was not a randomized trial, and data on ART initiation in asymptomatic adults with CD4+ counts >500 are less robust. In addition, this patient has exhibited behavior that raises questions about his ability to comply with ART. Therefore, rather than initiate ART at this time, you should educate the patient about the need to take better care of himself (i.e., to stop using IV drugs). You might also discuss the risks and benefits of ART initiation. Once this patient demonstrates that he can be compliant with HIV care, ART initiation should be strongly considered.

References

1. Kitahata MM et al. Effect of early vs. deferred antiretroviral therapy for HIV on survival. *N Engl J Med.* 2009;360(18):1815–1826.
2. When to Start Consortium. Timing of initiation of antiretroviral therapy in AIDS-free HIV-1-infected patients: a collaborative analysis of 18 HIV cohort studies. *Lancet.* 2009;373(9672):1352.
3. Cohen MS et al. Prevention of HIV-1 infection with early antiretroviral therapy. *N Engl J Med.* 2011;365(6):493.

4. SMART Study Group. CD4+ count-guided interruption of antiretroviral treatment. *N Engl J Med.* 2006;355(22):2283.

5. SMART Study Group. Major clinical outcomes in antiretroviral therapy (ART)-naive participants and in those not receiving ART at baseline in the SMART study. *J Infect Dis.* 2008;197(8):1133.

6. Günthard HF, Aberg JA, Eron JJ, Hoy JF, Telenti A, Benson CA, Burger DM, Cahn P, Gallant JE, Glesby MJ, Reiss P, Saag MS, Thomas DL, Jacobsen DM, Volberding PA; International Antiviral Society-USA Panel. Antiretroviral treatment of adult HIV infection: 2014 recommendations of the International Antiviral Society-USA Panel. *JAMA.* 2014 Jul 23–30;312(4):410–25.

SECTION 8

Cardiology

25

Statins in Healthy Patients with an Elevated C-Reactive Protein

The JUPITER Trial

MICHAEL E. HOCHMAN

> In this randomized trial of [healthy patients] with elevated levels of high-sensitivity C-reactive protein, rosuvastatin significantly reduced the incidence of major cardiovascular events, despite the fact that nearly all study participants had [normal lipid levels].
>
> —RIDKER ET AL.[1]

Research Question: Are statins effective in healthy patients with elevated C-reactive protein levels but without hyperlipidema?[1]

Funding: AstraZeneca.

Year Study Began: 2003

Year Study Published: 2008

Study Location: 1,315 sites in 26 countries.

Who Was Studied: Men ≥50 and women ≥60 without prior cardiovascular disease and with an LDL cholesterol <130 mg/dL and a high-sensitivity

C-reactive protein (CRP) ≥2.0 mg/L. The median CRP of patients screened for the trial was 1.9 mg/L (i.e., slightly more than half of all screened patients had a CRP below the level necessary for trial inclusion).

Who Was Excluded: Patients with a triglyceride level ≥500, those with previous or current use of lipid-lowering medications, those with an elevated alanine aminotransferase, creatine kinase, or creatinine, those with diabetes or uncontrolled hypertension, and those with cancer in the 5 years prior to enrollment. In addition, patients who did not take more than 80% of prescribed placebo pills in a 4-week pilot study were excluded because these patients were unlikely to comply with the trial medications.

How Many Patients: 17,802

Study Overview: See Figure 25.1 for a summary of the study's design.

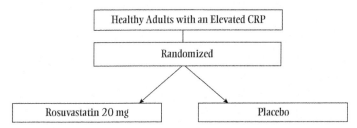

Figure 25.1 Summary of the Study Design.

Study Intervention: Patients were randomly assigned to receive either rosuvastatin 20 mg daily or placebo.

Follow-Up: Median 1.9 years.

Endpoints: Primary outcome: A composite of nonfatal myocardial infarctions, nonfatal strokes, hospitalizations for unstable angina, arterial revascularization, or cardiovascular death. Secondary outcome: Death from any cause.

RESULTS

- At baseline, the median LDL was 108 mg/dL in both groups; after 12 months, the median LDL was 55 mg/dL in the rosuvastatin group versus 110 mg/dL in the placebo group.

- At baseline, the median CRP was 4.2 mg/L in the rosuvastatin group and 4.3 mg/L in the placebo group; after 12 months, the median CRP was 2.2 mg/L in the rosuvastatin group versus 3.5 mg/dL in the placebo group.
- The incidence of diabetes was slightly higher during the study period in the rosuvastatin group than in the placebo group (3.0% versus 2.4%, $P = 0.01$).
- Rosuvastatin decreased cardiovascular events relative to placebo (see Table 25.1).

Table 25.1 SUMMARY OF KEY FINDINGS[a]

Outcome	Rosuvastatin Group	Placebo Group	*P* Value
Primary Composite Outcome	0.77	1.36	<0.00001
Myocardial Infarctions	0.17	0.37	0.0002
Stroke	0.18	0.34	0.002
Death	1.00	1.25	0.02

[a] Event rates are per 100 person-years, that is, the number of events that occurred for every 100 years of participant time. For example, 0.77 events per 100 person-years means that there were, on average, 0.77 events among 50 subjects who were each enrolled in the trial for 2 years.

Criticisms and Limitations: The absolute benefits of rosuvastatin were small: 95 patients would need to be treated for 2 years to prevent one cardiovascular event. Therefore, it is debatable whether the benefits of statins in healthy patients with an elevated CRP outweigh the potential long-term side effects.

In addition, it is unclear whether CRP levels should be used to help determine which patients should be treated with statins. It is possible that patients with normal CRP levels benefit just as much from statins as those with elevated levels.

Other Relevant Studies and Information:

- Other trials have also suggested a benefit of statins in patients without known cardiovascular disease; however, the absolute benefits of statins among such patients are small.[2,3]
- Guidelines from the American College of Cardiology and the American Heart Association (ACC/AHA) recommend statins for patients without known cardiovascular disease who have an LDL cholesterol ≥190 mg/dL and/or an estimated 10-year risk of cardiovascular disease ≥7.5%. These guidelines also recommend statins for patients with a history of cardiovascular disease or diabetes.[4]

- Guidelines from the Centers for Disease Control and the AHA, among other organizations, indicate that CRP measurement may be considered among patients with an intermediate cardiovascular risk (10%–20% over 10 years) to help determine whether or not statins should be used.[5] However, guidelines from the US Preventive Services Task Force do not recommend measuring CRP levels to help assess cardiovascular risk.[6]

Summary and Implications: Statin therapy reduced cardiovascular events in healthy patients with elevated CRP levels and normal lipids. However, the absolute benefits were small. The study did not assess whether CRP measurement is important for determining which patients should receive statins. Guidelines recommend statins for patients without known cardiovascular disease who have an LDL cholesterol ≥190 mg/dL and/or an estimated 10-year risk of cardiovascular disease ≥7.5%.

CLINICAL CASE: STATINS IN HEALTHY PATIENTS WITH AN ELEVATED C-REACTIVE PROTEIN

Case History:
A 70-year-old woman with a history of hypertension and tobacco use visits your clinic for a routine visit. She has a total cholesterol of 180, an HDL of 48, and an LDL of 120. Based on the results of JUPITER, should she be started on a statin?

Suggested Answer:
JUPITER demonstrated a small but significant benefit of statin therapy among patients without known cardiovascular disease and a CRP ≥2.0 mg/L. Because only patients with an elevated CRP level were included, the study did not evaluate the effectiveness of statins in other patients like the one in this vignette.

You might consider testing this patient's CRP. However, based on her age and risk factors, her calculated 10-year risk for cardiovascular disease is approximately 20%. Based on the guidelines from the ACC/AHA, it would be reasonable to consider statin therapy for her. Still, the absolute benefits of such therapy are likely to be small, and if she preferred not to take an additional medication it also would be reasonable to defer therapy.

References

1. Ridker PM et al. Rosuvastatin to prevent vascular events in men and women with elevated C-reactive protein. *N Engl J Med.* 2008;359(21):2195–2207.
2. Taylor F et al. Statins for the primary prevention of cardiovascular disease. *Cochrane Database Syst Rev.* 2013;1:CD004816.
3. Ray KK et al. Statins and all-cause mortality in high-risk primary prevention: a meta-analysis of 11 randomized controlled trials involving 65,229 participants. *Arch Intern Med.* 2010;170(12):1024.
4. Stone NJ et al. 2013 ACC/AHA Guideline on the Treatment of Blood Cholesterol to Reduce Atherosclerotic Cardiovascular Risk in Adults: a report of the American College of Cardiology/American Heart Association Task Force on Practice Guidelines. *J Am Coll Cardiol.* 2014;63:2889–2934.
5. Pearson TA et al. Markers of inflammation and cardiovascular disease: application to clinical and public health practice: a statement for healthcare professionals from the Centers for Disease Control and Prevention and the American Heart Association. *Circulation.* 2003;107(3):499.
6. US Preventive Services Task Force. Using nontraditional risk factors in coronary heart disease risk assessment: US Preventive Services Task Force recommendation statement. *Ann Intern Med.* 2009;151(7):474.

26

The Scandinavian Simvastatin Survival Study (4S)

WILLIAM BUTRON

> Simvastatin produced highly significant reductions in the risk of death and morbidity in patients with coronary heart disease . . . relative to patients receiving standard care.
> —SCANDINAVIAN SIMVASTATIN SURVIVAL STUDY GROUP[1]

Research Question: Do patients with a history of coronary heart disease (CHD) and an elevated total cholesterol benefit from long-term treatment with simvastatin?[1]

Funding: Merck Research Laboratories, the maker of simvastatin.

Year Study Began: 1988

Year Study Published: 1994

Study Location: 94 clinical centers in Scandinavia.

Who Was Studied: Adults 35–70 years old with CHD, defined as a history of cardiac chest pain or acute myocardial infarction and a serum cholesterol between 5.5 and 8.0 mmol/L (~210–310 mg/dL) following an 8-week trial of lifestyle modification and a 2-week placebo run-in period.

Who Was Excluded: Patients with serum triglyceride >2.5 mmol/L (~220 md/dL) were excluded, along with patients who had a contraindication to the study drug or who were already receiving the study drug. Also excluded were patients with cardiac conditions such as Prinzmetal's angina; hemodynamically significant valvular heart disease; persistent atrial fibrillation; congestive heart failure (CHF) requiring treatment with digitalis, diuretics, or vasodilators; or a myocardial infarction within the past 6 months.

How Many Patients: 4,444

Study Overview: See Figure 26.1 for a summary of the study's design.

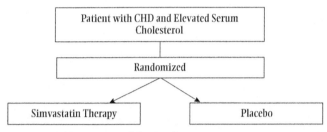

Figure 26.1 Summary of the Study Design.

Study Intervention: Patients in the simvastatin group were started on simvastatin 20 mg daily with regular follow-up. At the 12-week and 6-month visits, adjustments to the simvastatin dose were made. The dose could be increased to 40 mg or decreased to 10 mg based on the total serum cholesterol level. A total cholesterol level of 3.0–5.2 mmol/L (~115–200 mg/dL) was targeted. Patients in the control group received placebo therapy with mock dosing adjustments.

Follow-Up: Median of 5.4 years.

Endpoints: Primary outcome: Total mortality. Secondary outcomes: Coronary events, defined as coronary death, nonfatal myocardial infarction, or silent myocardial infarction confirmed by electrocardiogram; the need for coronary revascularization (coronary surgery or angioplasty); and cerebrovascular events.

RESULTS

- Baseline characteristics were similar between the two groups with an average age of 59 years and a mean serum cholesterol at baseline of 6.75 mmol/L (~260 mg/dL); 82% of participants were male.

- There was similar compliance to the study medication in both groups (87% in the simvastatin group versus 90% in the placebo group).
- Serum lipid improvement was greater in the simvastatin group compared to the placebo group, and at 1 year 72% of patients in the simvastatin group achieved the total cholesterol goal (Table 26.1).
- Total mortality was lower in the simvastatin group compared to the placebo group; this difference was driven predominantly by a reduction in cardiovascular mortality (Table 26.2).
- There were reductions in all types of atherosclerotic events in the simvastatin group versus the placebo group (Table 26.2).
- Prespecified stratified analyses revealed that the benefits of simvastatin were more pronounced in men versus women.

Table 26.1 CHANGE IN SERUM LIPIDS

	Simvastatin Group	Placebo Group
Total Cholesterol	−25%	+1%
LDL	−35%	+1%
Triglycerides	−10%	+7%
HDL	+8%	+1%

Table 26.2 SUMMARY OF KEY FINDINGS

	Simvastatin Group	Placebo Group	P Value
Total Mortality	8.2%	11.5%	0.0003
Cardiovascular Mortality	6.1%	9.3%	not reported
Noncardiovascular Mortality	2.1%	2.2%	not reported
Major Coronary Events	19.0%	28.0%	<0.00001
Coronary Surgery or Angioplasty	11.3%	17.2%	not reported
Cerebrovascular Events	2.7%	4.3%	not reported

Criticisms and Limitations: Patients were only invited to participate in this trial if they were compliant with placebo therapy during a run-in phase. This eligibility process selected for compliant and motivated patients. In a real-world setting, patient compliance with statin therapy would likely be lower, and thus the benefits of statin therapy would likely be lower.

The proportion of participants taking aspirin was lower than expected for this population (37% at the start of the trial and 55% at the end of follow-up). Among a study population with greater use of aspirin—which also protects against recurrent cardiovascular events—the benefits of statin therapy relative to placebo might have been less pronounced.

Additionally, nearly 80% of participants had a history of myocardial infarction, and thus the results may not be generalizable to patients with a history of angina but not myocardial infarction.

Other Relevant Studies and Information:

- Other trials also demonstrate the benefits of statin therapy for reducing all-cause and cardiovascular mortality among patients with established cardiovascular disease.[2]
- Statins have also been shown to be effective in the primary prevention of cardiovascular disease, though the absolute benefits are smaller for primary prevention (see Chapter 25 on the JUPITER trial).[3,4,5]
- Guidelines from the American College of Cardiology and American Heart Association recommend initiation of statin therapy in four high-risk groups: (1) patients with established atherosclerotic cardiovascular disease; (2) those with elevations in LDL ≥190 mg/dL, (3) those with diabetes and an LDL ≥70; and (4) those with a calculated 10-year risk of an atherosclerotic cardiovascular event >7.5% and an LDL ≥70.[6]

Summary and Implications: The 4S trial demonstrated a clear morbidity and mortality benefit from the use of statins in patients with established atherosclerotic cardiovascular heart disease and an elevated total cholesterol level. Statins are now recommended for all patients with established cardiovascular disease.

CLINICAL CASE: IMPACT OF STATIN THERAPY FOR PATIENTS WITH CHD

Case History:
A 65-year-old man with a history of two prior myocardial infarctions presents for a routine examination. He denies any cardiovascular symptoms, and he takes aspirin and blood pressure medications. You are surprised to note that he is not receiving statin therapy. His fasting lipid panel is notable for a total cholesterol level of 160 and an LDL of 90. Would you initiate a statin in this patient?

Suggested Answer:

The 4S trial demonstrated a benefit of statin therapy in patients with established cardiovascular disease and elevated lipid levels. The patient in this vignette has established cardiovascular disease; however, his lipid levels are not elevated. Still, because of strong evidence of benefit from statins for secondary cardiovascular prevention in other studies, guidelines from the American College of Cardiology and American Heart Association recommend initiation of statin therapy in all patients with established cardiovascular disease, regardless of lipid levels. Thus, it would be appropriate to suggest initiation of statin therapy in this patient.

References

1. Randomised trial of cholesterol lowering in 4,444 patients with coronary heart disease: the Scandinavian Simvastatin Survival Study (4S). *Lancet.* 1994;344:1383.
2. Wilt TJ et al. Effectiveness of statin therapy in adults with coronary heart disease. *Arch Intern Med.* 2004;164(13):1427.
3. Ridker PM et al. Rosuvastatin to prevent vascular events in men and women with elevated C-reactive protein. *N Engl J Med.* 2008;359(21):2195–2207.
4. Taylor F et al. Statins for the primary prevention of cardiovascular disease. *Cochrane Database Syst Rev.* 2013;1(1):CD004816. doi:10.1002/14651858. CD14004816.pub14651855.
5. Ray KK et al. Statins and all-cause mortality in high-risk primary prevention: a meta-analysis of 11 randomized controlled trials involving 65,229 participants. *Arch Intern Med.* 2010;170(12):1024.
6. Goff DC Jr et al. 2013 ACC/AHA guideline on the assessment of cardiovascular risk: a report of the American College of Cardiology/American Heart Association Task Force on Practice Guidelines. *Circulation.* 2014;129(25 Suppl 2):S49–73.

27

Choosing First-Line Therapy for Hypertension

The ALLHAT Trial

MICHAEL E. HOCHMAN

[The] results of ALLHAT indicate that thiazide-type diuretics should be considered first for pharmacologic therapy in patients with hypertension. They are unsurpassed in lowering [blood pressure], reducing clinical events, and tolerability, and they are less costly.
—THE ALLHAT INVESTIGATORS[1]

Research Question: What is the preferred first-line medication for the treatment of hypertension: thiazide diuretics or any of the more recently developed blood pressure medications?[1]

Funding: The National Heart, Lung, and Blood Institute.

Year Study Began: 1994

Year Study Published: 2002

Study Location: Approximately 600 general medicine and specialty clinics in the United States, Canada, Puerto Rico, and the Virgin Islands.

Who Was Studied: Adults ≥55 with stage 1 or stage 2 hypertension and at least one additional cardiovascular (CV) risk factor, including prior myocardial infarction or stroke, left ventricular hypertrophy, type 2 diabetes, current smoking, HDL cholesterol <35, or known atherosclerosis.

Who Was Excluded: Patients with a history of symptomatic heart failure, those with an ejection fraction <35%, and those with a serum creatinine >2 mg/dL.

How Many Patients: 33,357 (>42,000 patients were originally included; however, an arm of the trial involving patients receiving doxazosin was terminated early when it became clear that doxazosin was inferior to other study medications).

Study Overview: See Figure 27.1 for a summary of ALLHAT's design.

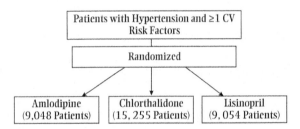

Figure 27.1 Summary of the Study Design.

- A disproportionate number of patients were assigned to the chlorthalidone arm because medications from this class (thiazide diuretics) were the established first-line treatment for hypertension at the time. Assigning more patients to the chlorthalidone arm allowed for greater statistical power for detecting differences between chlorthalidone and the other study medications.

Study Intervention: Patients were randomly assigned in a double-blinded fashion to receive either a thiazide diuretic (chlorthalidone, initially at a dose of 12.5 mg with a maximum dose of 25 mg); a calcium channel blocker (amlodipine, initially at a dose of 2.5 mg with a maximum dose of 10 mg); or an angiotensin-converting enzyme (ACE) inhibitor (lisinopril, initially at a dose of 10 mg with a maximum dose of 40 mg).

After being randomized, patients discontinued any prior antihypertensive medications and immediately began taking their assigned medication. The goal blood pressure for all patients was <140/90, and the study medications were titrated as needed to achieve this goal.

When the goal blood pressure could not be achieved with the study medication, additional open-label medications were added (these medications were added similarly in all trial arms).

Follow-Up: Mean of 4.9 years.

Endpoints: Primary outcome: A composite of fatal coronary heart disease (CHD) and nonfatal myocardial infarction. Secondary outcomes: Heart failure, stroke, and all-cause mortality.

RESULTS

- After five years, 68.2% of patients in the chlorthalidone group achieved the blood pressure goal, versus 66.3% in the amlodipine group ($P = 0.09$) and 61.2% in the lisinopril group ($P < 0.001$).
- Chlorthalidone was at least as effective as—and in some respects superior to—amlodipine and lisinopril in preventing cardiovascular disease (see Table 27.1).

Table 27.1 SUMMARY OF KEY FINDINGS[a]

Outcome	Chlorthalidone	Amlodipine	Lisinopril	P Value[b]
Heart Failure	7.7%	10.2%	8.7%	<0.001, <0.001
Stroke	5.6%	5.4%	6.3%	0.28, 0.02
All-Cause Mortality	17.3%	16.8%	17.2%	0.20, 0.90
Fatal CHD and Nonfatal Myocardial Infarction	11.5%	11.3%	11.4%	0.65, 0.81

[a] Rates are 6-year event rates per 100 persons.
[b] Chlorthalidone vs. amlodipine, chlorthalidone vs. lisinopril.

Criticisms and Limitations: The ALLHAT investigators chose to use chlorthalidone to represent thiazide diuretics because this was the best-studied agent in the class. However, the less potent hydrochlorothiazide is more commonly used in the United States. ALLHAT's findings may not be applicable to hydrochlorothiazide.

Other Relevant Studies and Information:

- An initial arm of ALLHAT involving doxazosin was terminated early when initial data indicated that chlorthalidone reduced the risk of cardiovascular events relative to doxazosin.[2]
- The ACCOMPLISH trial compared hydrochlorothiazide versus amlodipine (both in combination with benazepril) in patients with hypertension and high CV risk and showed amlodipine to be superior.[3] Many experts believe that the discrepancy between the results of ALLHAT and ACCOMPLISH is due to the fact that ALLHAT used chlorthalidone while ACCOMPLISH used hydrochlorothiazide. In addition, the dose of hydrochlorothiazide (12.5–25 mg) used in ACCOMPLISH is lower than some experts recommend.
- The 2014 Evidence-Based Guideline for the Management of High Blood Pressure in Adults recommends any of the following agents as first-line therapy for hypertension: ACE inhibitors, angiotensin receptor blockers (ARBs), calcium channel blockers (CCBs), or thiazide-type diuretics. The guidelines indicate that CCBs and thiazide-type diuretics are preferable for African Americans. Although thiazides were more effective than CCBs and ACE inhibitors with respect to some outcomes in ALLHAT, the guidelines cite similar outcomes with respect to overall mortality and coronary heart disease, and they thus conclude that any of these agents are appropriate first-line therapies.[4]

Summary and Implications: ALLHAT found that chlorthalidone, an inexpensive thiazide diuretic, is at least as effective as amlodipine and lisinopril as first-line therapy in high-risk patients with hypertension. Thiazide diuretics remain one of the preferred first-line medications for patients with hypertension.

CLINICAL CASE: CHOOSING FIRST-LINE THERAPY FOR HYPERTENSION

Case History:
A 60-year-old man with diabetes has been diagnosed with hypertension after repeated blood pressure measurements averaging 162/94. He reports feeling well. Routine laboratory tests are normal, except for the presence of moderate proteinuria.

Based on the results of ALLHAT, how should this patient be treated?

> **Suggested Answer:**
>
> ALLHAT established that a thiazide diuretic—chlorthalidone—is at least as effective as several other medications as first-line therapy in high-risk patients with hypertension. For this reason, thiazide diuretics are one of the preferred first-line medications for hypertension.
>
> The patient in this vignette has diabetic nephropathy (due to his proteinuria). In such patients, most experts would recommend an ACE inhibitor or ARB as first-line treatment for hypertension. Still, this patient has stage 2 hypertension (systolic blood pressure ≥160 or diastolic blood pressure ≥100) and thus multiple agents may be necessary as initial treatment. Chlorthalidone (which many experts believe to be the preferred thiazide diuretic) would be a good choice as a secondary agent.

References

1. ALLHAT Officers and Coordinators for the ALLHAT Collaborative Research Group. Major outcomes in high-risk hypertensive patients randomized to angiotensin-converting enzyme inhibitor or calcium channel blocker vs. diuretic: the antihypertensive and lipid-lowering treatment to prevent heart attack trial (ALLHAT). *JAMA.* 2002;288(23):2981–2997.
2. The ALLHAT Officers and Coordinators for the ALLHAT Collaborative Research Group. Major cardiovascular events in hypertensive patients randomized to doxazosin vs. chlorthalidone: the antihypertensive and lipid-lowering treatment to prevent heart attack trial (ALLHAT). *JAMA.* 2000;283:1967–1975.
3. Jamerson K et al. Benazepril plus amlodipine or hydrochlorothiazide for hypertension in high-risk patients. *N Engl J Med.* 2008;359(23):2417–2428.
4. James PA et al. 2014 evidence-based guideline for the management of high blood pressure in adults: report from the panel members appointed to the Eighth Joint National Committee (JNC 8). *JAMA.* 2014 Feb 5;311(5):507–520.

28

Rate Control versus Rhythm Control for Atrial Fibrillation

The AFFIRM Trial

MICHAEL E. HOCHMAN

[In older patients with atrial fibrillation and cardiovascular risk factors] the strategy of restoring and maintaining sinus rhythm [has] no clear advantage over the strategy of controlling the ventricular rate.
—THE AFFIRM INVESTIGATORS[1]

Research Question: Should patients with atrial fibrillation be managed with a strategy of rate control or rhythm control?[1]

Funding: The National Heart, Lung, and Blood Institute.

Year Study Began: 1997

Year Study Published: 2002

Study Location: 200 sites in the United States and Canada.

Who Was Studied: Adults with atrial fibrillation who were at least 65 or who had other risk factors for stroke. In addition, only patients likely to have recurrent atrial fibrillation requiring long-term treatment were eligible.

Who Was Excluded: Patients in whom anticoagulation was contraindicated.

How Many Patients: 4,060

Study Overview: See Figure 28.1 for a summary of AFFIRM's design.

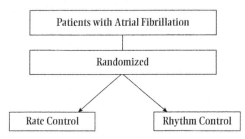

Figure 28.1 Summary of the Study Design.

Study Intervention: Patients in the rhythm-control group received antiarrhythmic drugs (most commonly amiodarone and/or sotalol) at the discretion of the treating physician. If needed, physicians could attempt to cardiovert patients to sinus rhythm. Anticoagulation with warfarin was encouraged but could be stopped at the physician's discretion if the patient remained in sinus rhythm for at least 4 (and preferably 12) consecutive weeks.

Patients in the rate-control group received beta blockers, calcium channel blockers, or digoxin at the discretion of the treating physician. The target heart rate was ≤80 beats per minute at rest and ≤110 beats per minute during a 6-minute walk test. All patients in the rate-control group received anticoagulation with warfarin.

Follow-Up: Mean of 3.5 years.

Endpoints: Primary outcome: All-cause mortality. Secondary outcomes: A composite of death, disabling stroke, disabling anoxic encephalopathy, major bleeding, and cardiac arrest; and hospitalizations.

RESULTS

- In the rate-control group, at the 5-year visit, 34.6% of patients were in sinus rhythm, and more than 80% of those in atrial fibrillation had adequate heart rate control.

- In the rhythm-control group, at the 5-year visit, 62.6% of patients were in sinus rhythm.
- After 5 years, 14.9% of patients in the rate-control group crossed over to the rhythm-control group, most commonly due to symptoms such as palpitations or episodes of heart failure.
- After 5 years, 37.5% of patients in the rhythm-control group crossed over to the rate-control group, most commonly due to an inability to maintain sinus rhythm or due to drug intolerance.
- Throughout the study, more than 85% of patients in the rate-control group were taking warfarin compared to approximately 70% of patients in the rhythm-control group; most strokes in both groups occurred among patients not receiving a therapeutic dose of warfarin.
- Patients in the rate-control group had fewer hospitalizations than those in the rhythm-control group and there was a nonsignificant trend toward lower mortality (see Table 28.1).

Table 28.1 SUMMARY OF KEY FINDINGS

Outcome	Rate-Control Group	Rhythm-Control Group	*P* Value
All-Cause Mortality	25.9%	26.7%	0.08
Composite of Death, Disabling Stroke, Disabling Anoxic Encephalopathy, Major Bleeding, and Cardiac Arrest	32.7%	32.0%	0.33
Hospitalizations	73.0%	80.1%	<0.001

Criticisms and Limitations: The trial did not include young patients without cardiovascular risk factors, especially those with paroxysmal atrial fibrillation, and therefore the results may not apply to these patients.

In addition, approximately half of the patients in the study had symptomatic episodes of atrial fibrillation less than once a month. It is possible that patients with more frequent or persistent symptoms would derive a benefit from rhythm control.

Other Relevant Studies and Information:

- A number of smaller randomized trials comparing rate control and rhythm control in patients with atrial fibrillation have come to similar conclusions as AFFIRM.[2-5]

- Trials comparing rate control with rhythm control in patients with atrial fibrillation and heart failure have also failed to show a benefit of rhythm control.[6,7]
- A recent observational study suggested lower long-term mortality with a rhythm-control strategy versus a rate-control strategy.[8] However, because this was not a randomized trial, the results are far from definitive and should not lead to a change in clinical practice.[9]
- Guidelines recommend rate control as the preferred initial strategy for treating older patients with paroxysmal, persistent, or permanent atrial fibrillation. However, rhythm control remains appropriate for certain patients such as those who remain symptomatic despite rate-control therapy and younger patients who are symptomatic.[10]

Summary and Implications: In high-risk patients with atrial fibrillation, a strategy of rate control is at least as effective as a strategy of rhythm control. Rhythm control does not appear to obviate the need for anticoagulation. Because the medications used for rate control are usually safer than those used for rhythm control, rate control is the preferred strategy for treating most high-risk patients with atrial fibrillation. These findings do not necessarily apply to younger patients without cardiovascular risk factors who were not included in AFFIRM, however.

CLINICAL CASE: RATE VERSUS RHYTHM CONTROL IN ATRIAL FIBRILLATION

Case History:
A 75-year-old woman with diabetes and hypertension is noted on routine examination to have an irregular heart rate of approximately 120 beats per minute. She denies chest pain, shortness of breath, and other concerning symptoms. An EKG confirms a diagnosis of atrial fibrillation.

Based on the results of AFFIRM, how should this patient be treated?

Suggested Answer:
AFFIRM showed that rate control is at least as effective as rhythm control for managing atrial fibrillation. Because the medications used for rate control are usually safer than those used for rhythm control, rate control is generally the preferred strategy for managing the condition.

The patient in this vignette is typical of patients included in AFFIRM. Thus, she should be treated initially with a rate-control strategy (beta blockers are frequently used as first-line agents). In the unlikely event that this patient's heart rate could not be controlled or if she were to develop bothersome symptoms that did not improve with a rate-control strategy, rhythm control might be considered. In addition, this patient should receive anticoagulation to reduce her risk for stroke.

References

1. The AFFIRM Investigators. A comparison of rate control and rhythm control in patients with atrial fibrillation. *N Engl J Med.* 2002;347(23):1825–1833.
2. Van Gelder IC et al. A comparison of rate control and rhythm control in patients with recurrent persistent atrial fibrillation. *N Engl J Med.* 2002;347(23):1834–1840.
3. Hohnloser SH et al. Rhythm or rate control in atrial fibrillation: Pharmacological Intervention in Atrial Fibrillation (PIAF); a randomised trial. *Lancet.* 2000;356(9244):1789–1794.
4. Carlsson J et al. Randomized trial of rate-control vs. rhythm-control in persistent atrial fibrillation: the Strategies of Treatment of Atrial Fibrillation (STAF) study. *J Am Coll Cardiol.* 2003;41(10):1690–1696.
5. Opolski G et al. Rate control vs rhythm control in patients with nonvalvular persistent atrial fibrillation: the results of the Polish How to Treat Chronic Atrial Fibrillation (HOT CAFE) Study. *Chest.* 2004;126(2):476–486.
6. Roy D et al. Rhythm control vs. rate control for atrial fibrillation and heart failure. *N Engl J Med.* 2008;358(25):2667–2677.
7. Kober L et al. Increased mortality after dronedarone therapy for severe heart failure. *N Engl J Med.* 2008;358(25):2678–2687.
8. Ionescu-Ittu R et al. Comparative effectiveness of rhythm control vs. rate control drug treatment effect on mortality in patients with atrial fibrillation. *Arch Intern Med.* 2012;172(13):997.
9. Dewland TA, Marcus GM. Rate vs. rhythm control in atrial fibrillation: can observational data trump randomized trial results? *Arch Intern Med.* 2012;172(13):983.
10. January CT et al. 2014 AHA/ACC/HRS Guideline for the Management of Patients with Atrial Fibrillation: executive summary: a report of the American College of Cardiology/American Heart Association Task Force on Practice Guidelines and the Heart Rhythm Society. *Circulation.* 2014 Apr 10. [Epub ahead of print].

29

Initial Treatment of Stable Coronary Artery Disease

The COURAGE Trial

MICHAEL E. HOCHMAN

> Our findings [confirm] . . . that [percutaneous coronary intervention] can be safely deferred in patients with stable coronary artery disease, even in those with extensive, multivessel involvement and inducible ischemia, provided that intensive, multifaceted medical therapy is instituted and maintained.
>
> —BODEN ET AL.[1]

Research Question: Should patients with stable coronary artery disease (CAD) be managed initially with medical therapy versus percutaneous coronary intervention (PCI)?[1]

Funding: The Department of Veterans Affairs, and the Canadian Institutes of Health Research.

Year Study Began: 1999

Year Study Published: 2007

Study Location: 50 centers in the United States and Canada.

Who Was Studied: Adults with stable CAD as defined by either a ≥70% stenosis in at least one proximal coronary artery along with objective evidence of ischemia on an EKG or stress test, or a ≥80% stenosis in a proximal coronary artery and classic angina symptoms. Patients with multivessel disease were included.

Who Was Excluded: Patients with class IV angina, a markedly positive stress test (i.e., substantial ST depression or hypotension during stage 1 of Bruce protocol stress test), refractory heart failure, ejection fraction <30%, or coronary anatomy unsuitable for PCI.

How Many Patients: 2,287

Study Overview: See Figure 29.1 for a summary of COURAGE's design.

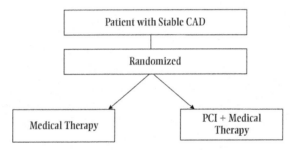

Figure 29.1 Summary of the Study Design.

Study Interventions: Patients in the medical therapy group received aspirin (or clopidogrel in patients with an aspirin allergy), lisinopril or losartan, and the following anti-ischemic medications: metoprolol, amlodipine, and isosorbide mononitrate, alone or in combination. In addition, patients received simvastatin alone or in combination with ezetimibe for a goal low-density lipoprotein (LDL) of 60–85, a goal high-density lipoprotein (HDL) >40, and a goal triglycerides <150.

Patients in the PCI group underwent target lesion PCI along with additional revascularization as clinically appropriate. Patients in this group also received aspirin and clopidogrel, and the same anti-ischemic medications, blood pressure medications, and lipid management as patients in the medical therapy group.

Follow-Up: Median of 4.6 years.

Endpoints: Primary outcome: A composite of death from any cause and non-fatal myocardial infarction. Secondary outcomes: Angina symptom control and quality of life.[2]

RESULTS

- 88% of patients in the PCI group successfully received stents.
- 70% of subjects in both groups achieved an LDL <85, while 65% achieved a systolic blood pressure <130.
- Patients in the medical therapy group and PCI group had similar rates of death or myocardial infarction (see Table 29.1).
- Initially, patients in the PCI group had a small but significant improvement in angina symptoms and quality of life. However, these differences were no longer present by the end of the study period.

Table 29.1 Summary of Key Findings[a]

Outcome	Medical Therapy Group	PCI Group	P Value
Death or Nonfatal Myocardial Infarction	18.5%	19.0%	0.62
Hospitalizations for Acute Coronary Syndrome	11.8%	12.4%	0.56
Additional Revascularization Necessary[b]	32.6%	21.1%	<0.001

[a] Estimated 4.6-year cumulative event rates.
[b] The need for PCI and/or coronary artery bypass surgery in the medical therapy group or the need for a repeat of these procedures in the PCI group.

Criticisms and Limitations: Drug-eluting stents—which now are in common use—were not used in the PCI group until the final 6 months of the study. Some argue that COURAGE should be repeated using drug-eluting stents (though it is not clear that drug-eluting stents lead to better outcomes than do bare metal stents).

Other Relevant Studies and Information:

- Other studies comparing PCI with medical therapy have come to similar conclusions as the COURAGE trial.[3,4,5]

- The BARI-2D trial showed similar outcomes among patients with diabetes who were treated with medical therapy versus revascularization (either PCI or coronary artery bypass surgery at their physicians' discretion), though a subgroup analysis suggested that patients who received coronary artery bypass surgery had the best outcomes.[6]
- The STICH trial, which compared coronary artery bypass surgery with medical therapy in patients with coronary artery disease and an ejection fraction ≤35%, found that the two treatments led to similar mortality rates.[7]
- Patients with high-risk coronary artery disease—such as ≥50% stenosis in the left main coronary artery, severe three-vessel disease, or proximal disease of the left anterior descending artery—are likely to benefit from coronary artery bypass surgery.[8]
- There also may be a subset of patients with stable coronary artery disease who benefit from initial revascularization with stenting: a recent study suggested a benefit of PCI versus optimal medical therapy among patients with severe stenosis identified using a technique called fractional flow reserve;[9] this finding will require further evaluation, however.[10]
- Based on the results of COURAGE and other studies, major guidelines recommend initial medical management for most patients with stable angina, except those with high-risk criteria, with PCI reserved for those who have bothersome symptoms despite medical therapy.[11]
- Despite the results of the COURAGE trial and the guidelines noted above, many US patients with stable coronary disease do not receive a trial of optimal medical therapy before undergoing PCI.[12]

Summary and Implications: In most patients with stable coronary artery disease (including multivessel disease), medical therapy and percutaneous coronary intervention (PCI) lead to similar outcomes. For most patients, medical therapy is an appropriate—and generally preferable—initial management strategy, though a substantial proportion of medically managed patients may ultimately require PCI to treat refractory symptoms. Certain high-risk patients, such as those with a markedly positive stress test or severe symptoms, should receive initial PCI, however.

CLINICAL CASE: INITIAL TREATMENT OF STABLE CORONARY ARTERY DISEASE

Case History:

A 62-year-old man visits your clinic to review the results of his recent stress test. For the past year, he has noted substernal discomfort when climbing steps or walking up hills. The pain is relieved with rest. Aside from a daily baby aspirin, your patient does not take any medications.

During the stress test, your patient was able to exercise for 6 minutes and achieved 7 METS of activity. His peak heart rate was 148 beats per minute. Toward the end of the test, he developed the same substernal chest discomfort that he typically experiences. He also developed lateral ST depressions on EKG. A repeat stress test with nuclear imaging confirmed reversible ischemia in the territory of the left circumflex coronary artery. In addition, the cardiac function appeared to be mildly impaired (ejection fraction 45%–50%).

You explain to your patient that he has stable coronary artery disease. Based on the results of the COURAGE trial, how would you treat him?

Suggested Answer:

The COURAGE trial suggests that, for most patients with stable coronary artery disease, medical therapy is an appropriate—and generally preferable—initial management strategy.

The patient in this vignette is typical of those included in the COURAGE trial. He doesn't have any of the high-risk features that might suggest that he would benefit from immediate revascularization. Thus he would be a good candidate for medical management. Should his symptoms worsen in the future despite optimal medical therapy, he might require revascularization to help manage his symptoms. However, revascularization is not necessary at this point.

References

1. Boden WE et al. Optimal medical therapy with or without PCI for stable coronary disease. *N Engl J Med.* 2007;356(15):1503–1516.
2. Weintraub WS et al. Effect of PCI on quality of life in patients with stable coronary disease. *N Engl J Med.* 2008;358:677.
3. Tirkalinos TA et al. Percutaneous coronary interventions for non-acute coronary artery disease: a quantitative 20-year synopsis and a network meta-analysis. *Lancet.* 2009;373(9667):911.

4. Stergiopoulos K, Brown DL. Initial coronary stent implantation with medical therapy vs. medical therapy alone for stable coronary artery disease: meta-analysis of randomized controlled trials. *Arch Intern Med.* 2012;172(2):312–319.

5. Bangalore S, Pursnani S, Kumar S, Bagos PG. Percutaneous coronary intervention versus optimal medical therapy for prevention of spontaneous myocardial infarction in subjects with stable ischemic heart disease. *Circulation.* 2013;127(7):769.

6. BARI 2D Study Group. A randomized trial of therapies for type 2 diabetes and coronary artery disease. *N Engl J Med.* 2009;360(24):2503–2515.

7. Velazquez EJ et al. Coronary-artery bypass surgery in patients with left ventricular dysfunction. *N Engl J Med.* 2011;364:1607–1616.

8. Hillis LD et al. 2011 ACCF/AHA Guideline for Coronary Artery Bypass Graft Surgery: executive summary: a report of the American College of Cardiology Foundation/American Heart Association Task Force on Practice Guidelines. *Circulation.* 2011;124(23):2610.

9. De Bruyne B et al. Fractional flow reserve-guided PCI versus medical therapy in stable coronary disease. *N Engl J Med.* 2012;367(11):991.

10. Boden WE. Which is more enduring—FAME or COURAGE? *N Engl J Med.* 2012;367:11,1059–1061.

11. Levine GN et al. 2011 ACCF/AHA/SCAI Guideline for Percutaneous Coronary Intervention: executive summary: a report of the American College of Cardiology Foundation/American Heart Association Task Force on Practice Guidelines and the Society for Cardiovascular Angiography and Interventions. *Circulation.* 2011;124(23):2574.

12. Boden WB et al. Patterns and intensity of medical therapy in patients undergoing percutaneous coronary intervention. *JAMA.* 2011;305(18):1882–1889.

Early Invasive versus Conservative Management for Unstable Angina or Non-ST-Elevation Myocardial Infarction

The RITA 3 Trial

LAVANYA KONDAPALLI

For patients with unstable angina or non-ST-elevation myocardial infarction, at moderate risk, an interventional strategy is preferable to a strategy of ischemia-provoked revascularization.

—THE RITA 3 INVESTIGATORS[1]

Research Question: Do patients with unstable angina (UA) or non-ST-elevation myocardial infarction (NSTEMI) benefit from early invasive management with angiography followed by revascularization if appropriate?[1]

Funding: The British Heart Foundation, which received donations from Aventis Pharma.

Year Study Began: 1997

Year Study Published: 2002

Study Location: 45 hospitals in England and Scotland.

Who Was Studied: Patients with "suspected cardiac chest pain at rest" and at least one additional sign of coronary artery disease: (1) ECG with signs of ischemia, (2) pathologic Q waves suggesting past myocardial infarction, or (3) coronary artery disease on prior angiogram.

Who Was Excluded: Patients with likely myocardial infarction in whom invasive management was indicated, those with new Q waves, CK or CK-MB levels twice the upper limit of normal, myocardial infarction in the past 30 days, or percutaneous coronary intervention (PCI) in the past 12 months were excluded.

How Many Patients: 1,810

Study Overview: See Figure 30.1 for a summary of the RITA 3 design.

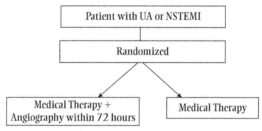

Figure 30.1 Summary of the Study Design.

Study Intervention: Patients in the optimal medical therapy group received anti-anginals at the discretion of the treating physician, including a beta blocker if not contraindicated. Aspirin, enoxaparin, and other antithrombotic agents (including glycoprotein IIb/IIIa inhibitors) were also administered at the discretion of the treating physician. Patients who continued to have severe anginal symptoms despite the above therapy, or in whom anti-anginal therapy could not be withdrawn, could be referred for coronary angiography.

Patients in the invasive group received optimal medical therapy as described above as well as coronary angiography "as soon as possible following randomization and ideally within 72 hours." Based on the results of angiography, the treating physician decided whether revascularization was indicated and, if so, whether PCI or coronary artery bypass grafting (CABG) should be utilized. When possible, revascularization procedures were performed during the initial hospital admission.

Follow-Up: Median of 2 years.

Endpoints: Primary endpoints: Combined rate of death, nonfatal myocardial infarction, or refractory angina at 4 months; and combined rate of death or nonfatal myocardial infarction at 1 year. Refractory angina was defined as chest pain during the index hospitalization requiring revascularization or readmission with ischemic chest pain.

RESULTS

- In the invasive group, angiography identified 78% of patients as having at least one significantly stenosed vessel. PCI was planned for 36% of patients in the invasive group and CABG for 22%; the rest received pharmacologic management only.
- The revascularization rate was 57% in the invasive group versus 28% in the conservative group (i.e., 28% of patients in the conservative therapy group were treated with revascularization).
- Rates of death, myocardial infarction, or refractory angina were lower in the invasive group versus the conservative therapy group at 4 months; this benefit was driven by a reduction in the rate of angina. Rates of death or myocardial infarction were similar between the groups at 1 year (see Table 30.1).

Table 30.1 Summary of Key Findings

Outcome	Invasive Group	Conservative Group	*P* Value
Death, Myocardial Infarction, or Refractory Angina at 4 Months	9.6%	14.5%	0.001
Death	2.9%	2.5%	0.61
Myocardial Infarction	3.4%	3.7%	0.68
Angina	4.4%	9.3%	<0.0001
Death or Myocardial Infarction at 1 Year	7.6%	8.3%	0.58
Death	4.6%	3.9%	0.50
Myocardial Infarction	3.8%	4.8%	0.29

Criticisms and Limitations: The primary benefit from an early invasive approach was a decrease in refractory angina. Though refractory angina was defined as possible cardiac chest pain with ECG changes, it is unclear whether treating physicians were sufficiently aggressive in the medical management of angina before reporting treatment failure.

Of the patients, 38% were women. A subgroup analysis among women showed the incidence of both co-primary endpoints was similar in the invasive group and in the medical therapy group. Therefore, it is unclear whether these study results are applicable to female patients.

Other Relevant Studies and Information:

- In a 5-year follow-up analysis of RITA 3, the invasive group had lower rates of death or nonfatal myocardial infarction (odds ratio 0.78, 95% CI 0.61–0.99, $P = 0.044$) and of cardiovascular death or nonfatal myocardial infarction ($P = 0.030$) than the medical therapy group. High-risk patients benefited the most from invasive therapy.[2]
- A meta-analysis of long-term outcomes in three trials of routine invasive therapy in UA/NSTEMI, including data from RITA 3, found reductions in cardiovascular death and nonfatal myocardial infarction at 5 years with the invasive strategy (hazard ratio 0.81, $P = 0.002$); the analysis showed an 11.1% absolute risk reduction in a subgroup analysis of high-risk patients.[3]
- Other randomized control trials have also shown benefit of an early invasive strategy over conservative medical therapy in treating UA and NSTEMI.[4,5]
- The American College of Cardiology/American Heart Association (ACC/AHA) guidelines give Class I recommendations to early invasive therapy in two groups of patients with UA/NSTEMI: (1) those with refractory angina or hemodynamic instability and (2) those with high risk of clinical events.[6]

Summary and Implications: Patients with UA or NSTEMI who were treated with early angiography and subsequent revascularization if appropriate had lower rates of cardiovascular events—mostly driven by a reduction in angina—than those treated conservatively after 4 months. After 5 years of follow-up, patients in the invasive group had lower rates of death and myocardial infarction. The ACC/AHA guidelines recommend that high-risk patients with UA/NSTEMI should be managed with an early invasive strategy.

CLINICAL CASE: EARLY INVASIVE VERSUS CONSERVATIVE MANAGEMENT OF UA/NSTEMI

Case History:

A 63-year-old male with known coronary artery disease, hypertension, and diabetes presents to the emergency department with an hour of stuttering chest pain. The pain originates in the center of his chest, radiates to his left arm, and comes and goes every 20 minutes. Vital signs are notable for a blood pressure of 95/60, and he reports that he did not take his antihypertensives today. Initial troponin is at the upper limit of normal. The ECG reveals T wave inversion in the anterior leads.

Based on the results of RITA 3, how should this patient be treated?

Suggested Answer:

This patient is suffering from an acute coronary syndrome and should receive aspirin, oxygen, and morphine for pain control. A right-sided ECG should be performed to exclude right-sided infarct, given the patient's hypotension before administering sublingual nitroglycerin. Heparin or enoxaparin should be initiated as well. Beta blockers should not be administered given the patient's hypotension.

Based on the results of RITA 3, this patient would also be a good candidate for cardiac catheterization. In the short term, he is likely to suffer less angina with an early invasive strategy, and in the long term he may be less likely to die or experience myocardial infarction. Because he is hemodynamically unstable (low blood pressure) he falls into a high-risk category and is thus a particularly good candidate for early intervention.

References

1. Fox KAA et al. Interventional versus conservative treatment for patients with unstable angina or non-ST-elevation myocardial infarction: The British Heart Foundation RITA 3 randomized trial. *Lancet.* 2002;360:743–751.
2. Fox KAA et al. Five year outcome of an interventional strategy in non-ST-elevation acute coronary syndrome: the British Heart Foundation RITA 3 randomized trial. *Lancet.* 2005;366:914–920.
3. Fox KA et al. Long term outcome of a routine versus selective invasive strategy in patients with non-ST-segment elevation acute coronary syndrome: a meta-analysis of individual patient data. *J Am Coll Cardiol.* 2010;55(22):2435–2445.
4. FRISC II Investigators. Invasive compared with non-invasive treatment in unstable coronary-artery disease: FRISC II prospective randomized multicenter study. *Lancet.* 1999;354:708–715.

5. Cannon CP et al. Comparison of early invasive and conservative strategies in patients with unstable coronary syndromes treated with glycoprotein IIb/IIIa inhibitor tirofiban. *NEJM*. 2001;344(25):1879–1887.

6. Jneid H et al. 2012 ACCF/AFA focused update of the guideline for the management of patients with unstable angina/non-ST-elevation myocardial infarction (updating the 2007 guideline and replacing the 2011 focused update): A report for the American College of Cardiology Foundation/American Heart Association task force on practice guidelines. *Circulation*. 2012;126:875–910.

31

Prophylactic Defibrillator Implantation in Patients with Low Ejection Fraction following Myocardial Infarction

The MADIT II Trial

JOSHUA R. THOMAS

> Our findings show that the implantation of a defibrillator improves survival in patients with a prior myocardial infarction and advanced left ventricular dysfunction.
>
> —MOSS ET AL.[1]

Research Question: Does implantation of a cardiac defibrillator device improve survival in patients with a history of myocardial infarction and reduced ejection fraction?[1]

Funding: Guidant Corporation, the maker of the defibrillator used in the trial.

Year Study Began: 1997

Year Study Published: 2002

Study Location: 71 centers in the United States and 5 in Europe.

Who Was Studied: Patients ≥21 years of age with a history of myocardial infarction at least 1 month prior to entry and an ejection fraction ≤30% documented within the previous 3 months.

Who Was Excluded: Patients with other FDA-approved indications for implantation of a defibrillator were excluded. Also excluded were those with New York Heart Association functional class IV heart failure at the time of enrollment, "advanced cerebrovascular disease," or a high likelihood of short-term mortality from noncardiac causes. Patients with coronary revascularization within 3 months or myocardial infarction within 1 month of enrollment were also excluded.

How Many Patients: 1,232

Study Overview: See Figure 31.1 for a summary of the study's design.

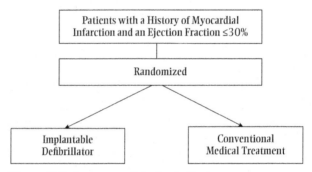

Figure 31.1 Summary of the Study Design.

Study Intervention: Patients randomized to receive a defibrillator had the device implanted in the usual manner with programming at the discretion of the treating physicians. Patients in the control group did not receive defibrillator implantation. Patients in both groups received other usual medical therapy at the discretion of the treating physicians.

Follow-Up: Mean of 20 months.

Endpoints: Primary outcome: All-cause mortality.

RESULTS

- Baseline characteristics were similar between the two groups with an average age of 65 years and a mean left ventricular ejection fraction of 23%; 85% of participants were men.

- Defibrillator therapy was associated with a reduction in all-cause mortality (Table 31.1; this reduction was also observed in subgroup analyses stratified by age, sex, ejection fraction, New York Heart Association class, and the QRS interval.
- No deaths occurred during defibrillator implantation; 2.5% of patients in the defibrillator group required surgical revision for lead problems or infection.

Table 31.1 SUMMARY OF KEY FINDINGS

Endpoint	Defibrillator Group	Control Group	*P* Value
Mortality	14.2%	19.8%	0.016

Criticisms and Limitations: The survival benefit associated with implantation of defibrillators was not evident until 9 months following implantation, a result that was also observed in the SCD-HeFT trial. Furthermore, there was a nonsignificant increase in heart failure observed in the defibrillator group (20% versus 15%, $P = 0.09$). Possible explanations for this finding include increased development of heart failure in patients whose survival was the result of defibrillator therapy, cardiac damage associated with defibrillator shocks, or an unknown consequence of implantation of the defibrillator.

Other Relevant Studies and Information:

- The original MADIT trial (MADIT I) demonstrated the benefit of defibrillator implantation in patients with a history of myocardial infarction, reduced ejection fraction, and evidence of nonsustained ventricular tachycardia and reproducible ventricular tachycardia.[2]
- The MUSTT and SCD-HeFT trials provide additional evidence of the benefit of implantable cardiac defibrillators in patients with a history of myocardial infarction and reduced ejection fraction.[3,4]
- The CABG Patch trial demonstrated that the implantation of defibrillators at the time of coronary artery bypass grafting among patients with coronary heart disease and a reduced ejection fraction did not reduce mortality;[5] similarly, implanting defibrillators within 40 days of myocardial infarction has not been associated with reduced mortality.[6,7]
- The American College of Cardiology/American Heart Association (ACC/AHA)/Heart Rhythm Society and European guidelines recommend implantation of a cardiac device in the following groups

of patients with a history of myocardial infarction: (1) those with an ejection fraction <30% and class I heart failure at least 40 days after the myocardial infarction; (2) those with an ejection fraction <35% and class II or III heart failure at least 40 days after the myocardial infarction; and (3) those with an ejection fraction <40% and inducible ventricular fibrillation or sustained ventricular tachycardia.[8]

Summary and Implications: MADIT II demonstrated that among patients with a history of myocardial infarction (excluding those with myocardial infarction within the previous month) and an ejection fraction ≤30%, implantation of a defibrillator leads to a reduction in mortality. Implantable defibrillators are now recommended among patients with a history of myocardial infarction and an ejection fraction <30% or with class II or III heart failure and ejection fraction <35%. The guidelines specify that implantation should be delayed at least 40 days following myocardial infarction in these groups due to evidence suggesting a lack of benefit when implanted within the first 40 days.

CLINICAL CASE: PROPHYLACTIC IMPLANTATION OF A CARDIAC DEFIBRILLATOR IN A PATIENT FOLLOWING MYOCARDIAL INFARCTION WITH A LOW EJECTION FRACTION

Case History:
A 58-year-old man presents for an episode of chest pain that occurred 1 week ago. He did not seek medical attention until now because he felt he could "just get through it." An ECG is done showing Q-waves that were not present on prior examinations. A subsequent echocardiogram shows an ejection fraction of 25%. The patient is otherwise asymptomatic.

Based on the results of the MADIT II trial, how should this patient be treated?

Suggested Answer:
Based on the clinical history, the patient appears to have experienced a myocardial infarction and now presents approximately 1 week later with a reduced ejection fraction. He should immediately receive appropriate medical care following myocardial infarction, including antiplatelet therapy, statins, antihypertensives, and an assessment of his coronary arteries.

> With respect to the decision of whether or not to implant a defibrillator, guidelines recommend waiting for a minimum of 40 days following myocardial infarction to assess ejection fraction and determine the need for an implantable defibrillator. This is due to data suggesting a lack of benefit with implantation within 40 days of myocardial infarction.
>
> If, on repeat examination at least 40 days after the likely event, the patient demonstrates an ejection fraction <30%, he would be a candidate for implantation of a defibrillator.

References

1. Moss AJ et al. Prophylactic implantation of a defibrillator in patients with myocardial infarction and reduced ejection fraction. *N Engl J Med*. 2002;346:877.
2. Moss AJ et al. Improved survival with an implanted defibrillator in patients with coronary disease at high risk for ventricular arrhythmia. Multicenter Automatic Defibrillator Implantation Trial Investigators. *N Engl J Med*. 1996;335:1933.
3. Buxton AE et al. A randomized study of the prevention of sudden death in patients with coronary artery disease. Multicenter Unsustained Tachycardia Trial Investigators. *N Engl J Med*. 1999;341:1882.
4. Bardy GH et al. Amiodarone or an implantable cardioverter-defibrillator for congestive heart failure. *N Engl J Med*. 2005;352:225.
5. Bigger JT Jr. Prophylactic use of implanted cardiac defibrillators in patients at high risk for ventricular arrhythmias after coronary-artery bypass graft surgery. Coronary Artery Bypass Graft (CABG) Patch Trial Investigators. *N Engl J Med*. 1997;337:1569.
6. Hohnloser SH et al. Prophylactic use of an implantable cardioverter-defibrillator after acute myocardial infarction. *N Engl J Med*. 2004;351:2481.
7. Steinbeck G et al. Defibrillator implantation early after myocardial infarction. *N Engl J Med*. 2009;361:1427.
8. Epstein AE et al. ACC/AHA/HRS 2008 Guidelines for Device-Based Therapy of Cardiac Rhythm Abnormalities: a report of the American College of Cardiology/ American Heart Association Task Force on Practice Guidelines (Writing Committee to Revise the ACC/AHA/NASPE 2002 Guideline Update for Implantation of Cardiac Pacemakers and Antiarrhythmia Devices): developed in collaboration with the American Association for Thoracic Surgery and Society of Thoracic Surgeons. *Circulation*. 2008;117:e350.

32

Captopril in Patients with Left Ventricular Dysfunction after Myocardial Infarction

The SAVE Trial

VIMAL RAMJEE

> We demonstrated in this study that long-term therapy with captopril in survivors of acute myocardial infarction with depressed left ventricular ejection fraction but without overt heart failure resulted in reductions in both total and cardiovascular mortality.
>
> —THE SAVE INVESTIGATORS[1]

Research Question: Does captopril reduce morbidity and mortality in patients with left ventricular dysfunction after a myocardial infarction?[1]

Funding: The Bristol-Myers Squibb Institute for Pharmaceutical Research.

Year Study Began: 1987

Year Study Published: 1992

Study Location: 112 hospitals in the United States and Canada.

Who Was Studied: Adults aged 21 to 79 years who survived the first 3 days after a myocardial infarction and had a left ventricular ejection fraction of ≤40% on radionucleotide ventriculography.

Who Was Excluded: Patients with an "unstable" post–myocardial infarction course, a contraindication to angiotensin-converting enzyme (ACE) inhibitors, symptomatic heart failure, hypertension requiring treatment with ACE inhibitors, a serum creatinine >2.5 mg/dL, or "other conditions believed to limit survival."

How Many Patients: 2,231

Study Overview: See Figure 32.1 for a summary of SAVE's design.

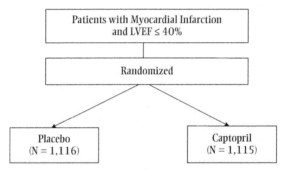

Figure 32.1 Summary of the Study Design.

Study Intervention: Patients in the captopril group were initiated on captopril 12.5 mg three times a day between 3 and 16 days following a myocardial infarction. A lower dose of 6.25 mg three times a day was permitted in patients who experienced a substantial decrease in blood pressure after receiving the initial dose. The target dose for the in-hospital phase was 25 mg three times daily. Following discharge, this dose was gradually increased to 50 mg three times daily as tolerated.

Follow-Up: Mean of 3.5 years.

Endpoints: All-cause mortality; cardiovascular mortality; and cardiovascular morbidity defined as severe congestive heart failure (CHF) or recurrent myocardial infarction (fatal or nonfatal).

RESULTS:

- There was no significant difference in baseline characteristics between the two groups with a mean age of 59 years and a mean ejection fraction of 31%.

- Blood pressure increased in both groups within 3 months, more so in the placebo versus captopril group ($P < 0.001$ for both systolic and diastolic).
- At 4 years, there was a significant reduction in all-cause and cardiovascular mortality and cardiovascular morbidity with captopril compared to placebo (Table 32.1).
- The therapeutic benefit of captopril persisted in subgroup analyses involving age, sex, history of myocardial infarction, ejection fraction, and Killip class (a scale used to predict 30-day mortality for a patient suffering an acute myocardial infarction; higher scores portend worse outcomes).
- There was no between-group difference in mortality from noncardiac causes.
- A subgroup analysis showed a disproportionate benefit of captopril in men relative to women (relative risk reduction for all-cause mortality of 2% in women versus 22% in men).

Table 32.1 SUMMARY OF KEY FINDINGS

Outcome	Captopril Group	Placebo Group	Relative Risk Reduction	*P* Value
All-Cause Mortality	20.4%	24.6%	19%	0.019
Cardiovascular Mortality	16.9%	21.0%	21%	0.014
Cardiovascular Morbidity				
CHF Resistant to Diuretics and Digoxin	10.6%	16.0%	37%	<0.001
CHF Hospitalization	13.8%	17.2%	22%	0.019
Recurrent Myocardial Infarction	11.9%	15.2%	25%	0.015

Criticisms and Limitations: The trial did not include adults older than 79 years, limiting generalizability to adults of advanced age.

Other Relevant Studies and Information:

- A number of other randomized controlled trials comparing ACE inhibitors to placebo in patients after a myocardial infarction have had findings consistent with SAVE.[2,3,4]
- While individual trials studying *early* post–myocardial infarction ACE inhibitor therapy (initiation within 24 hours) have yielded contradictory findings,[5,6] large meta-analyses advocate for early

initiation in selected patients—particularly those with high-risk characteristics.[7]

- Major guidelines now recommend ACE inhibitor therapy for patients following acute myocardial infarction who have a reduced ejection fraction. Guidelines also recommend consideration of ACE inhibitors following myocardial infarction for patients with preserved ejection fraction, particularly in those with high-risk features.[8]

Summary and Implications: In patients with left ventricular dysfunction after a myocardial infarction, the initiation of an ACE inhibitor provides significant mortality and morbidity benefit. ACE inhibitors are now recommended for all patients following myocardial infarction with a reduced ejection fraction, and they should also be considered in patients with a preserved ejection fraction following myocardial infarction, particularly in those with high-risk features.

CLINICAL CASE: ACE INHIBITORS POST–MYOCARDIAL INFARCTION

Case History:
A 63-year-old man with hypertension, diabetes, and hyperlipidemia presents to the ER with chest pain and is found to have a non-ST-elevation myocardial infarction. Cardiac catheterization shows near total occlusion of the mid-left anterior descending artery, and a drug-eluting stent is placed. In the intensive care unit five days later, an echocardiogram shows an ejection fraction of 30%. On examination, he is cold and his blood pressure is 77/32. He has no new complaints.

Based on the results of SAVE, how should this patient be treated?

Suggested Answer:
SAVE showed that the initiation of an ACE inhibitor 3 to 16 days after a myocardial infarction provided significant mortality and morbidity benefits. However, the trial excluded patients with post–myocardial infarction instability, or an absolute or relative contraindication of ACE inhibitors.

The patient in this vignette would have been excluded from the SAVE trial on the basis of his hypotension, qualifying as post–myocardial infarction instability and/or a contraindication to ACE inhibitor treatment. In this case, it would be safest to ensure that this patient's blood pressure improves before initiating an ACE inhibitor. Otherwise, he does have high-risk features that would warrant therapy as soon as it is safely possible.

References

1. The SAVE Investigators. Effect of captopril on morbidity and mortality in patients with left ventricular dysfunction after myocardial infarction. *N Engl J Med*. 1992 Sep 3;327(10):669–677.
2. The SOLVD Investigators. Effect of enalapril on survival in patients with reduced left ventricular ejection fractions and congestive heart failure. *N Engl J Med*. 1991;325:293–302.
3. The CONSENSUS Trial Study Group. Effects of enalapril on mortality in severe congestive heart failure: results of the Cooperative North Scandinavian Enalapril Survival Study (CONSENSUS). *N Engl J Med*. 1987;316:1429–1435.
4. Acute Infarction Ramipril Efficacy (AIRE) Study Investigators. Effect of ramipril on mortality and morbidity of survivors of acute myocardial infarction with clinical evidence of heart failure. *Lancet*. 1993;342(8875):821–828.
5. Swedberg K et al. Effects of the early administration of enalapril on mortality in patients with acute myocardial infarction—results of the Cooperative New Scandinavian Enalapril Survival Study II (CONSENSUS II). *N Engl J Med*. 1992;327:678–684.
6. Gruppo Italiano per lo Studio della Sopravvivenza nell'infarto Miocardico. GISSI-3: effects of lisinopril and transdermal glyceryl trinitrate singly and together on 6-week mortality and ventricular function after acute myocardial infarction. *Lancet*. 1994;343:1115–1122.
7. Oxenham H, Sharpe N. Angiotensin-converting enzyme inhibitor after myocardial infarction. *J Am Coll Cardiol*. 2000;36(7):2054–2055.
8. Anderson J et al. ACC/AHA 2007 guidelines for the management of patients with unstable angina/non-ST-elevation myocardial infarction: a report of the American College of Cardiology/American Heart Association Task Force on Practice Guidelines (Writing Committee to revise the 2002 Guidelines for the Management of Patients with Unstable Angina/Non-ST-Elevation Myocardial Infarction): developed in collaboration with the American College of Emergency Physicians, American College of Physicians, Society for Academic Emergency Medicine, Society for Cardiovascular Angiography and Interventions, and Society of Thoracic Surgeons. *J Am Coll Cardiol*. 2007;50:e1. www.acc.org/qualityand-science/clinical/statements.htm

33

Spironolactone in Advanced Heart Failure

The RALES Trial

VIMAL RAMJEE

[In patients with New York Heart Association (NYHA) class III or IV systolic heart failure] the addition of spironolactone to a standard heart failure regimen improved survival and reduced rates of hospitalization for heart failure.

—THE RALES INVESTIGATORS[1]

Research Question: Does the addition of spironolactone to standard heart failure therapy improve survival among patients with NYHA class III or IV systolic heart failure?[1]

Funding: G. D. Searle & Company (now a part of Pfizer), which manufactures spironolactone.

Year Study Began: 1995

Year Study Published: 1999

Study Location: 195 sites in 15 countries.

Who Was Studied: Adults with NYHA class III or IV heart failure at the time of enrollment with a left ventricular ejection fraction ≤35% measured within the previous 6 months. In addition, patients were required to have had NYHA class IV heart failure within 6 months of enrollment. All patients were managed with diuretics and an ACE inhibitor (if tolerated) prior to entering the trial.

Who Was Excluded: Patients with valvular heart disease unrelated to left ventricular heart failure and amenable to surgical correction and those with a history of or planned heart transplantation were excluded. Also excluded were patients with congenital heart disease, unstable angina, liver or kidney disease, cancer, or other serious illnesses other than heart failure. Patients with serum potassium >5 mmol/L or already on a potassium-sparing diuretic were also excluded.

How Many Patients: 1,663

Study Overview: See Figure 33.1 for a summary of the RALES design.

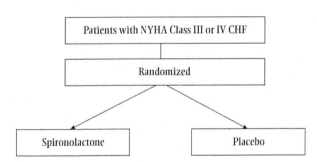

Figure 33.1 Summary of the Study Design.

Study Intervention: Patients were randomized to receive either spirono-lactone 25 mg once daily or a placebo pill. The spironolactone dose could be increased to 50 mg daily if symptoms of heart failure persisted after 8 weeks without hyperkalemia, or reduced to 25 mg every other day if hyper-kalemia developed. Similar adjustments could also be made in the placebo group.

Follow-Up: Mean of 2 years.

Endpoints: Primary outcome: All-cause mortality. Secondary outcomes: Cardiac death, hospitalization for cardiac cause, and change in NYHA class.

RESULTS

- There was no significant difference in baseline characteristics between the groups with an average age of 65 years; 73% of patients were male.
- There was a significant reduction in all-cause and cardiac mortality in the spironolactone group, with significant reductions in cardiac death from both progressive heart failure and sudden cardiac death (Table 33.1).
- There were significantly fewer hospitalizations for heart failure in the spironolactone group compared to the placebo group (Table 33.1).
- During the study period, more patients in the spironolactone group showed improvements in their NYHA class (41% versus 33%, $P < 0.001$).
- There was a small but significant increase in serum creatinine (median increase 0.05–0.10 mg/dL) and serum potassium (0.30 mmol/L) in the spironolactone group, but there were no significant differences in episodes of severe hyperkalemia between the groups.
- More men in the spironolactone group experienced gynecomastia (10% versus 1%, $P < 0.001$), causing more men in the spironolactone group to drop out of the study (10 versus 1, $P = 0.006$).

Table 33.1 SUMMARY OF KEY FINDINGS

Outcome	Placebo	Spironolactone	P Value
All-Cause Mortality	46%	35%	<0.001
Cardiac Death	37%	27%	<0.001
Death from Progression of Heart Failure	22%	15%	<0.001
Sudden Cardiac Death	13%	10%	0.02
Hospitalization for Cardiac Cause	40%	32%	<0.001

Criticisms and Limitations: Only patients with advanced heart failure were included in the study, and the results may not apply to patients with less severe versions of the disease. In addition, only patients with systolic heart failure were included and the results may not apply to patients with diastolic heart failure. There was also a low rate of beta blocker use (10%–11%) among study patients. It is possible that the impact of spironolactone is more modest among patients on beta blockers—which are now the standard of care for patients with systolic heart failure. Lastly, though patients with creatinine up to 2.5 mg/dL were eligible for enrollment, few participants with serum creatinine close to this threshold were enrolled, raising questions about the safety of introducing aldosterone antagonists in patients with advanced kidney disease.

Other Relevant Studies and Information:

- The EPHESUS trial[2] demonstrated a significant mortality benefit and reduction in hospitalizations with eplerenone (another potassium-sparing diuretic similar to spironolactone) in patients with a recent myocardial infarction and an ejection fraction ≤40%.
- The EMPHASIS-HF trial[3] showed that eplerenone reduced all-cause mortality and cardiac death among patients with mild congestive heart failure (NYHA class II).
- American College of Cardiology/American Heart Association (ACC/ AHA) guidelines recommend the addition of low-dose aldosterone antagonists in patients with severe or moderately severe symptomatic heart failure.[4]

Summary and Implications: In patients with NYHA class III or IV heart failure, the addition of spironolactone to standard heart failure therapy significantly reduced all-cause mortality, cardiac mortality, progression of heart failure, and hospitalization for heart failure. Spironolactone therapy was associated with modest elevations in serum creatinine and potassium levels. Patients with advanced heart failure without contraindications (advanced renal insufficiency or hyperkalemia) should be considered for spironolactone therapy.

CLINICAL CASE: SPIRONOLACTONE VERSUS PLACEBO IN HEART FAILURE

Case History:

A 52-year-old woman with ischemic cardiomyopathy (LVEF 30%), hypertension, and renal insufficiency presents for a routine follow-up. She has been coming to the clinic for 5 months, and during this time she has started several medications to treat her heart failure. She shows you her medication list, which includes metoprolol 25 mg twice a day, furosemide 40 mg daily, lisinopril 40 mg daily, and isosorbide dinitrate 10 mg three times a day. She tells you that she has been well but is still only able to walk one to two blocks before feeling short of breath and fatigued.

Her vitals are blood pressure of 100/63, a heart rate of 58, a respiratory rate of 14, a temperature of 98.9°F, and oxygen saturation of 98% on room air. Labs from the prior week show a creatinine of 1.4 mg/dL (her baseline is 1.3 mg/dL) and a potassium level of 4.8 mmol/L.

Based on the results of RALES, how should this patient be treated?

Suggested Answer:

RALES showed that for patients with NYHA class III or IV heart failure, spironolactone had a substantial mortality benefit and led to improvements in functional status.

This patient would likely benefit from the addition of spironolactone 25 mg daily. A close follow-up with a basic metabolic panel to reassess her creatinine level and potassium level would be prudent to ensure that she is tolerating the medication, particularly since she has an elevated creatinine and a potassium in the upper range of normal. If the patient tolerates spironolactone 25 mg daily, the dose could be titrated up to 50 mg daily.

References

1. Pitt B et al. The effect of spironolactone on morbidity and mortality in patients with severe heart failure. Randomized Aldactone Evaluation Study Investigators. *NEJM.* 1999;341(10):709–717.

2. Pitt B et al. Eplerenone, a selective aldosterone blocker, in patients with left ventricular dysfunction after myocardial infarction. *NEJM.* 2003;348(14):1309–1321. doi:10.1056/NEJMoa030207.

3. Zannad F et al. Eplerenone in patients with systolic heart failure and mild symptoms. *NEJM.* 2011;364(1):11–21. doi:10.1056/NEJMoa1009492.

4. Jessup M et al. 2009 focused update: ACCF/AHA Guidelines for the Diagnosis and Management of Heart Failure in Adults: a report of the American College of Cardiology Foundation/American Heart Association Task Force on Practice Guidelines: developed in collaboration with the International Society for Heart and Lung Transplantation. *Circulation.* 2009;119(14):1977–2016.

34

The African American Heart Failure Trial (A-HeFT)

MICHAEL E. HOCHMAN

> Our finding of the efficacy of isosorbide dinitrate plus hydralazine in black patients provides strong evidence that this therapy can slow the progression of heart failure. A future strategy would be to identify genotypic and phenotypic characteristics that would transcend racial or ethnic categories to identify a population with heart failure in which there is an increased likelihood of a favorable response to such therapy.
> —TAYLOR ET AL.[1]

Research Question: Is the combination of isosorbide dinitrate plus hydralazine effective for managing advanced heart failure in African Americans?[1]

Funding: NitroMed Pharmaceuticals.

Year Study Began: 2001

Year Study Published: 2004

Study Location: 161 centers in the United States.

Who Was Studied: African Americans ≥18 with New York Heart Association class III or IV heart failure (patients with heart failure symptoms with minimal exertion or at rest). Patients were required to have a depressed ejection fracture (≤35% or <45% with a severely dilated left ventricle). In addition, patients were required to be on appropriate heart failure therapy (e.g., angiotensin-converting enzyme [ACE] inhibitors, beta blockers, etc.).

The authors chose to study African Americans because retrospective studies had previously suggested that African Americans may respond particularly well to isosorbide dinitrate/hydralazine. In addition, African Americans have historically been underrepresented in cardiovascular research.

Who Was Excluded: Patients with a recent cardiovascular event, clinically significant valvular disease, symptomatic hypotension, or another illness likely to result in death during the study period.

How Many Patients: 1,050

Study Overview: See Figure 34.1 for a summary of A-HeFT's design.

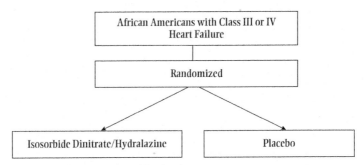

Figure 34.1 Summary of the Study Design.

Study Intervention: Patients in the isosorbide dinitrate/hydralazine group initially received a tablet containing 20 mg of isosorbide dinitrate and 37.5 mg of hydralazine, which they were instructed to take three times daily. If tolerated, the dose was titrated up to two tablets three times daily. Patients in the placebo group received a placebo tablet that was administered according to the same protocol.

Follow-Up: Mean of 10 months.

Endpoints: Primary outcome: A composite score incorporating death, a first hospitalization for heart failure, and change in the quality of life.

RESULTS

- The trial was stopped early after it became clear that mortality rates were higher in the placebo group (see Table 34.1).
- 47.5% of patients in the isosorbide dinitrate/hydralazine group reported headaches compared with 19.2% in the placebo group.
- 29.3% of patients in the isosorbide dinitrate/hydralazine group reported dizziness compared with 12.3% in the placebo group.
- The mean systolic blood pressure in the isosorbide dinitrate/hydralazine group dropped by 1.9 mm Hg, while the mean systolic blood pressure increased by 0.8 mm Hg in the placebo group.

Table 34.1 SUMMARY OF KEY FINDINGS

Outcome	Isosorbide Dinitrate/ Hydralazine Group	Placebo Group	P Value
Death	6.2%	10.2%	0.02
First Hospitalization for Heart Failure	16.4%	24.4%	0.001
Change in Quality of Life[a]	−5.6	-2.7	0.02
Composite Score[b]	−0.1	-0.5	0.01

[a] Quality of life was assessed using the Minnesota Living with Heart Failure Questionnaire. A lower score indicates a higher quality of life, that is, patients in the isosorbide dinitrate/hydralazine group reported a higher quality of life.
[b] A higher composite score indicates a better outcome, that is, patients in the isosorbide dinitrate/hydralazine group had better outcomes.

Criticisms and Limitations: A-HeFT only included patients with advanced heart failure; whether isosorbide dinitrate/hydralazine is effective among patients with less severe disease is unclear.

Patients in the isosorbide dinitrate/hydralazine group experienced a considerably higher rate of headaches and dizziness compared to patients in the placebo group, highlighting the need to use the medications cautiously.

Other Relevant Studies and Information:

- The V-HeFT I trial showed that isosorbide dinitrate/hydralazine is superior to placebo among men with heart failure who were not taking ACE inhibitors.[2]

- The V-HeFT II trial showed that the ACE inhibitor enalapril is superior to isosorbide dinitrate/hydralazine among men with heart failure.[3]
- Guidelines from the American College of Cardiology/American Heart Association recommend a combination of nitrate and hydralazine therapy for African American patients with moderate or severe symptoms of heart failure despite standard therapy with ACE inhibitors, beta blockers, and diuretics.[4]

Summary and Implications: The A-HeFT trial showed that isosorbide dinitrate/hydralazine, when added to standard heart failure therapy, improves outcomes in African Americans with New York Heart Association class III or IV heart failure and a reduced ejection fraction. A-HeFT is also significant because it focused on African American patients, who historically have been underrepresented in medical research.

CLINICAL CASE: ISOSORBIDE DINITRATE/ HYDRALAZINE FOR AFRICAN AMERICANS WITH HEART FAILURE

Case History:
A 66-year-old white man with New York Heart Association class IV heart failure (symptoms at rest) and an ejection fraction of 30% presents to your office for assistance in managing his symptoms. He reports taking lisinopril, carvedilol, spironolactone, amlodipine, furosemide, aspirin, atorvastatin, citalopram, gabapentin, and lorazepam. On exam, his heart rate is 72 and his blood pressure is 130/84. His lungs are clear and he has 1–2+ lower extremity edema.

Based on the results of A-HeFT, would you make any adjustments to this patient's medications to improve his heart failure therapy?

Suggested Answer:
The A-HeFT trial demonstrated that isosorbide dinitrate/hydralazine, when added to standard heart failure therapy, improves outcomes in African Americans with New York Heart Association class III or IV heart failure and a reduced ejection fraction. Except for the fact that he is white, the patient in this vignette is typical of patients included in the trial. While one might argue that the results should not be applied to this patient because he is white, African American patients are frequently treated based on results of research

that disproportionately involves white patients. For this reason, the author of this book believes that the results of A-HeFT should be applied to this patient, that is, he should be a candidate for isosorbide dinitrate/hydralazine.

On the other hand, however, the patient in this vignette is currently receiving 10 medications, and adding isosorbide dinitrate/hydralazine would further complicate his already complex medication regimen. Therefore, rather than adding isosorbide dinitrate/hydralazine, it might be preferable to increase the dose of another medication (perhaps the lisinopril) to help manage his symptoms. If isosorbide dinitrate/hydralazine is added, the patient should be monitored very carefully for hypotension and other side effects (headaches and dizziness).

References

1. Taylor AL et al. Combination of isosorbide dinitrate and hydralazine in blacks with heart failure. *N Engl J Med.* 2004;351(20):2049–2056.
2. Cohn JN et al. Effect of vasodilator therapy on mortality in chronic congestive heart failure: results of a Veterans Administration cooperative study. *N Engl J Med.* 1986;314(24):1547–1552.
3. Cohn JN et al. A comparison of enalapril with hydralazine-isosorbide dinitrate in the treatment of chronic congestive heart failure. *N Engl J Med.* 1991;325(5):303–310.
4. Hunt SA et al. 2009 focused update incorporated into the ACC/AHA 2005 Guidelines for the Diagnosis and Management of Heart Failure in Adults: a report of the American College of Cardiology Foundation/American Heart Association Task Force on Practice Guidelines: developed in collaboration with the International Society for Heart and Lung Transplantation. *Circulation.* 2009;119(14):e391.

35

Intra-Aortic Balloon Support for Myocardial Infarction with Cardiogenic Shock

The IABP-SHOCK II Trial

STEVEN D. HOCHMAN

> Use of intraaortic balloon counterpulsation [in patients with myocardial infarction and cardiogenic shock], as compared with conventional therapy, did not reduce 30-day mortality.
>
> —THIELE ET AL.[1]

Research Question: Among patients with cardiogenic shock due to acute myocardial infarction, does intra-aortic balloon support, in addition to standard care, improve survival?[1]

Funding: Multiple German governmental agencies, the University of Leipzig, and Maquet Cardiopulmonary and Teleflex Medical, both makers of intra-aortic balloon pumps.

Year Study Began: 2009

Year Study Published: 2012

Study Location: 37 centers in Germany.

Who Was Studied: Patients with acute myocardial infarction (ST-elevation or non-ST elevation) complicated by cardiogenic shock with planned revascularization. Cardiogenic shock was defined as either:

- Systolic blood pressure <90 mm Hg for at least 30 minutes, or
- The combination of dependence on "catecholamines to maintain systolic blood pressure >90 mm Hg," pulmonary congestion, and clinical or laboratory evidence of organ damage (e.g., altered mental status or elevated serum lactate)

Who Was Excluded: Patients older than 90 years, those with "mechanical causes of cardiogenic shock (e.g., papillary muscle rupture)," those who had "undergone resuscitation for >30 minutes" or with shock lasting for >12 hours before enrollment, those with no intrinsic heart activity, and those "in a coma with fixed dilation of pupils." Also excluded were those with other comorbidities with a high risk of mortality within 6 months.

How Many Patients: 600

Study Overview: See Figure 35.1 for a summary of the study design.

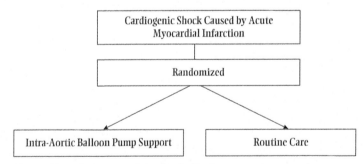

Figure 35.1 Summary of the Study Design.

Study Intervention: Patients randomized to intra-aortic balloon pump support received the device either before or after the planned revascularization procedure at the discretion of the treating physician. Pump support was maintained until patients had achieved a systolic blood pressure >90 mm Hg for at least 30 minutes without catecholamine support, at which point the pump was weaned.

Patients in the routine-care group did not receive intra-aortic balloon pump support unless they developed mechanical complications leading to pump failure (e.g., ventricular wall or papillary muscle rupture).

Patients in both groups underwent revascularization (percutaneous coronary intervention [PCI] or coronary artery bypass grafting [CABG]) and additional care at the discretion of the treating team.

Follow-Up: 30 days

Endpoints: Primary outcome: All-cause mortality. Secondary outcomes: Reinfarction and stroke.

RESULTS

- Baseline characteristics were similar between groups with a median age of 70 years; 69% of participants were male.
- 10% of patients randomized to the routine-care group received intra-aortic balloon pumps (in most cases, these pumps were placed against study protocol); 4.3% of patients randomized to the intra-aortic balloon support group did not receive the device.
- There was no difference in 30-day mortality between groups in the intention-to-treat or per-protocol analyses (Table 35.1).
- Results were consistent across all prespecified subgroups, including patients with an ST segment elevation myocardial infarction (STEMI) versus a non-STEMI, and those who received balloon pumps before versus after revascularization.

Table 35.1 SUMMARY OF KEY FINDINGS

Variable	IABP Group	Routine-Care Group	P Value
30-Day Mortality (Intention-to-Treat)	39.7%	41.3%	0.69
30-Day Mortality (Per-Protocol)	37.5%	41.4%	0.35
Reinfarction	3.0%	1.3%	0.16
Stroke in Hospital	0.7%	1.7%	0.28

Criticisms and Limitations: A large number (10%) of patients in the routine-care group ended up receiving balloon pumps against the study protocol, which may have affected the study results. However, the per-protocol analysis (which analyzes patients according to the treatment they received rather than the treatment they were assigned to) also failed to demonstrate a benefit with balloon pumps.

The overall mortality rate for patients in this study was 40%, which is relatively low for patients with cardiogenic shock and acute myocardial infarction. Therefore, it is possible that the results of this study do not apply to sicker or more rapidly deteriorating patients.

Other Relevant Studies and Information:

- A follow-up analysis from this study showed similar mortality rates in the two groups after one year (52% in the IABP group versus 51% in the routine-care group).[2]
- A 2009 meta-analysis of observational studies involving more than 10,000 patients failed to demonstrate a mortality benefit from intra-aortic balloon pumps in cardiogenic shock.[3]
- The 2013 guidelines from the American College of Cardiology/ American Heart Association (ACC/AHA) do not recommend the routine use of intra-aortic balloon pump. However, the guidelines state that balloon pumps "can be useful for patients with cardiogenic shock after STEMI who do not quickly stabilize with pharmacologic therapy" (such patients were not well represented in IABP-SHOCK II).[4]

Summary and Implications: IABP-SHOCK II demonstrated similar mortality rates among patients with myocardial infarction and cardiogenic shock who did and did not receive intra-aortic balloon support. The ACC/AHA guidelines state that balloon pumps may be useful for patients "who do not quickly stabilize with pharmacological therapy" (a group that was not well represented in IABP-SHOCK II) but do not recommend their routine use for patients with myocardial infarction and cardiogenic shock.

CLINICAL CASE: CARDIOGENIC SHOCK FOLLOWING MYOCARDIAL INFARCTION

Case History:
A 68-year-old man with a history of diabetes, dyslipidemia, and hypertension is brought in by ambulance after collapsing while walking with his wife. On presentation to the emergency room, his blood pressure is 78/40 with a heart rate of 120. The ECG shows ST-elevations in leads II, III, and aVF. How should this patient be managed?

Suggested Answer:

This patient most likely has an inferior wall ST-elevation myocardial infarction and cardiogenic shock. Early revascularization with PCI or CABG is the mainstay of therapy, and the patient should be taken for revascularization as soon as possible. The patient is hemodynamically unstable and should be resuscitated immediately with fluids and pharmacologic therapy. IABP-SHOCK II suggests that this patient is unlikely to benefit from intra-aortic balloon pump therapy. However, if he remains hemodynamically unstable despite other therapies including vasopressors, the ACC/AHA guidelines indicate that balloon pump therapy may be useful (such patients were not well represented in IABP-SHOCK II).

References

1. Thiele H et al. Intraaortic balloon support for myocardial infarction with cardiogenic shock. *N Engl J Med*. 2012;367:1287.
2. Thiele H et al. Intra-aortic balloon counterpulsation in acute myocardial infarction. *Lancet*. 2013 Nov;382(9905):1638–1645.
3. Sjauw KD et al. A systematic review and meta-analysis of intra-aortic balloon pump therapy in ST-elevation myocardial infarction: should we change the guidelines? *Eur Heart J*. 2009;30:459.
4. O'Gara PT et al. 2013 ACCF/AHA guideline for the management of ST-elevation myocardial infarction: a report of the American College of Cardiology Foundation/American Heart Association Task Force on Practice Guidelines. *Circulation*. 2013; 127(4): e362–425.

Pulmonary and Critical Care Medicine

36

Intensive versus Conventional Glucose Control in Critically Ill Patients

The NICE-SUGAR Study

KRISTOPHER SWIGER

> In this ... trial involving adults in the intensive care unit, we found that intensive glucose control, as compared to conventional glucose control, increased the absolute risk of death ...
>
> —THE NICE-SUGAR INVESTIGATORS[1]

Research Question: Does an aggressive blood glucose target (81–108 mg/dL) in critically ill patients result in different outcomes compared to a more conventional target (<180 mg/dL)?[1]

Funding: The Australian National Health and Medical Research Council, the Health Research Council of New Zealand, and the Canadian Institute for Health Research, all public granting agencies.

Year Study Began: 2004

Year Study Published: 2009

Study Location: Medical and surgical intensive care units (ICUs) at 42 hospitals (38 academic centers and 4 community hospitals) in Australia, Canada, New Zealand, and the United States.

Who Was Studied: Medical and surgical ICU patients older than 18 years with an expected ICU stay of at least 3 days and not expected to be eating by mouth within 48 hours.

Who Was Excluded: Patients whose treating physicians objected to enrollment and those who could not personally or through a surrogate provide informed consent. Also excluded were patients with an admitting diagnosis of diabetic ketoacidosis or hyperosmolar state. Lastly, patients with a history of hypoglycemic episodes or risk factors predisposing to hypoglycemia were excluded.

How Many Patients: 6,104

Study Overview: See Figure 36.1 for a summary of the study's design.

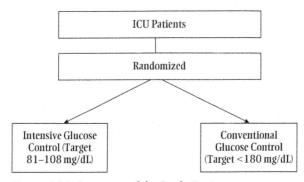

Figure 36.1 Summary of the Study Design.

Study Intervention: Patients were randomly assigned to intensive glucose control, with a target blood glucose of 81 to 108 mg/dL, or to conventional glucose control, with a target blood glucose <180 mg/dL. In both groups, blood glucose was sampled from arterial catheters (if possible) and measured with glucose meters, blood gas analyzers, or central laboratory assays. Insulin was administered by intravenous infusion. The trial intervention was discontinued when patients were eating or discharged from the ICU, but it was resumed if patients were readmitted to the ICU within 90 days.

Follow-Up: 90 days

Endpoints: Primary outcome: Death from any cause within 90 days. Secondary and tertiary outcomes: Cause-specific mortality, duration of mechanical ventilation, duration of renal-replacement therapy, new onset organ failure, and length of hospital and ICU stay.

RESULTS

- Patients in the intensive therapy group were significantly more likely to receive insulin and had lower average blood sugar levels than those in the conventional group (Table 36.1).
- At 90 days, patients in the intensive therapy group had significantly higher mortality compared to those in the conventional group (Table 36.1).
- Patients in the intensive therapy group experienced more episodes of severe hypoglycemia compared to those in the conventional group (Table 36.1).
- There were no major differences observed in prespecified subgroup analyses comparing surgical versus nonsurgical patients, those with and without diabetes, those with and without severe sepsis, and those with and without APACHE scores over 25.
- Patients in the intensive therapy group had higher mortality from all cardiovascular causes compared to the control group (41.6% versus 35.8%, $P = 0.02$). However, there was no difference in other specific causes of mortality.
- The duration of mechanical ventilation or renal replacement therapy, onset of organ failure, and length of stay in the ICU and hospital were similar between the two groups.

Table 36.1 SUMMARY OF KEY FINDINGS

Variable	Intensive Glucose Control	Conventional Glucose Control	P Value
Treated with Insulin	97.2%	69.0%	<0.001
Mean Daily Insulin Dose	50.2 units/day	16.9 units/day	<0.001
Time-Weighted Average Blood Glucose	118 mg/dL	145 mg/dL	<0.001
90-Day Mortality	27.5%	24.9%	0.02
Severe Hypoglycemia	6.8%	0.5%	<0.001

Criticisms and Limitations: The study has been criticized for its unblinded design and its subjective inclusion criteria of patients expected to be in the ICU for at least 3 days. Additionally, NICE-SUGAR chose different target glucose levels than previous studies, making comparisons with other studies difficult. Furthermore, a significant portion of patients allocated to the intensive control group did not achieve the glucose treatment targets.

Other Relevant Studies and Information:

- Prior to NICE-SUGAR, two trials compared intensive glucose control (target 80–110 mg/dL) to conventional control (target 180–200 mg/dL) in surgical[2] and medical[3] ICU patients. The surgical trial found a one-year reduction in the mortality rate in the intensively managed group (4.6% versus 8.0%, $P < 0.04$). However, no difference in mortality was found among medical ICU patients.
- The 2012 Surviving Sepsis Guidelines from the Society of Critical Care Medicine recommends a glycemic target of <180 mg/dL in patients with severe sepsis.[4]
- The American Association of Clinical Endocrinologists and American Diabetes Association recommend initiating insulin therapy in critically ill patients with a blood glucose greater than 180 mg/dL and with a target blood sugar of 140–180 mg/dL.[5]

Summary and Implications: NICE-SUGAR demonstrated that intensive glucose lowering among ICU patients to achieve a glucose goal of less than 108 mg/dL increased mortality compared to a conventional blood sugar target of <180 mg/dL. Although controversy persists about the optimal blood sugar targets for ICU patients, particularly surgical patients, most guidelines now recommend conservative targets of <180 mg/dL.

CLINICAL CASE: GLUCOSE MONITORING IN THE ICU

Case History:
A 56-year-old man is admitted to the medical ICU for hypoxic respiratory failure from healthcare-associated pneumonia. He is placed on the mechanical ventilator. He has a known history of type II diabetes mellitus and takes insulin at home. You note his admission blood glucose is 150 mg/dL. What blood glucose goal should you strive for while he remains in the ICU?

Suggested Answer:
The NICE-SUGAR trial demonstrated that intensive glucose control with a target blood glucose of 81–108 mg/dL increased all-cause mortality relative to a more conservative target of <180 mg/dL. This patient is typical of those included in NICE-SUGAR, and it would be appropriate to target a blood glucose <180 mg/dL rather than a more aggressive target.

References

1. Finfer S et al. Intensive versus conventional glucose control in critically ill patients. *N Engl J Med*. 2009;360(13):1283–1297.
2. Van den Berghe G et al. Intensive insulin therapy in critically ill patients. *N Engl J Med*. 2001;345:1359.
3. Van den Berghe G et al. Intensive insulin therapy in the medical ICU. *N Engl J Med*. 2006;354:449.
4. Dellinger RP et al. Surviving sepsis campaign: international guidelines for management of severe sepsis and septic shock: 2012. *Crit Care Med*. 2013;41(2):580–637.
5. Moghissi ES et al. American Association of Clinical Endocrinologists and American Diabetes Association consensus statement on inpatient glycemic control. *Endocr Pract*. 2009;15(4):353–369.

Red Cell Transfusion in Critically Ill Patients

The TRICC Trial

MICHAEL E. HOCHMAN

> Our findings indicate that the use of a threshold for red-cell transfusion as low as 7.0 [grams] of hemoglobin per deciliter ... was at least as effective as and possibly superior to a liberal transfusion [threshold of 10.0 g/dL] in critically ill patients.
>
> —HÉBERT ET AL.[1]

Research Question: When should patients in the intensive care unit (ICU) with anemia receive red cell transfusions?[1]

Funding: The Medical Research Council of Canada and an unrestricted grant from the Bayer Corporation (the Bayer grant was given after funding had been secured from the Medical Research Council of Canada).

Year Study Began: 1994

Year Study Published: 1999

Study Location: 25 ICUs in Canada.

Who Was Studied: Adults in medical and surgical ICUs with a hemoglobin (hgb) <9.0 g/dL, and who were clinically euvolemic.

Who Was Excluded: Patients with considerable active blood loss (e.g., gastro-intestinal bleeding leading to a drop in hgb of at least 3.0 points in the preceding 12 hours), chronic anemia (documented hgb <9.0 g/dL at least 1 month before admission), and those who were pregnant.

How Many Patients: 838

Study Overview: See Figure 37.1 for a summary of TRICC's design.

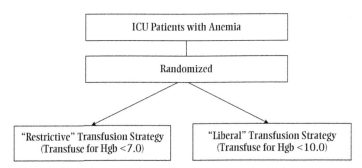

Figure 37.1 Summary of the Study Design.

Study Intervention: Non-leukocyte-reduced red cells were transfused according to the above thresholds and were given one unit at a time. After each transfusion, the patient's hemoglobin was measured and additional transfusions were given as needed.

Follow-Up: 30 days.

Endpoints: Primary outcome: 30-day mortality. Secondary outcomes: 60-day mortality, multiorgan failure.

RESULTS

- Approximately 30% of patients had a primary respiratory diagnosis; 20% had a primary cardiac diagnosis; 15% had a primary gastrointestinal illness; and 20% had a primary diagnosis of trauma.
- Patients in the "restrictive" group received an average of 2.6 units of blood during the trial, compared to an average of 5.6 units in the liberal group.
- The average daily hgb in the "restrictive" group was 8.5 versus 10.7 in the "liberal" group.

- As indicated in Table 37.1, there was no significant difference in 30-day mortality between patients in the "restrictive" versus "liberal" groups. However, in a subgroup analysis involving younger and healthier patients 30-day mortality rates were significantly lower in the "restrictive" group.
- In another subgroup analysis involving patients with cardiac disease, there was no significant difference in 30-day mortality between patients in the "restrictive" versus "liberal" groups. However, patients with acute coronary syndromes had nonsignificantly improved outcomes with the "liberal" transfusion strategy.[2]
- Cardiac events (pulmonary edema and myocardial infarction) were significantly more common in the "liberal" group.

Table 37.1 SUMMARY OF KEY FINDINGS

Outcome	"Restrictive" Group	"Liberal" Group	P Value
30-Day Mortality	18.7%	23.3%	0.11
60-Day Mortality	22.7%	26.5%	0.23
Multiorgan Failure[a]	5.3%	4.3%	0.36

[a] More than three failing organs.

Criticisms and Limitations: A disproportionate number of patients with severe cardiac disease did not participate in the trial because their physicians chose not to enroll them. In addition, the red cells used in this trial were not leukocyte-reduced. Some centers now routinely use leukocyte-reduced blood, which may be associated with few transfusion-related complications.

Other Relevant Studies and Information:

- A review of trials comparing restrictive versus liberal transfusion strategies concluded that "existing evidence supports the use of restrictive transfusion [strategies] in patients who are free of serious cardiac disease." However, "the effects of conservative transfusion [strategies] on functional status, morbidity and mortality, particularly in patients with cardiac disease, need to be tested in further large clinical trials."[3]
- Trials have supported the use of a restrictive transfusion strategy in patients undergoing elective coronary artery bypass surgery,[4] patients who have undergone surgery for a hip fracture,[5] patients with recent traumatic brain injuries,[6] and children in the ICU.[7]

- A restrictive transfusion strategy (hgb threshold ≤7 g/dL) proved superior to a liberal strategy (hgb threshold ≤ 9 g/dL) among patients with acute upper gastrointestinal bleeding.[8]
- A small trial involving elderly patients admitted to the hospital with a hip fracture compared a liberal transfusion strategy (hgb threshold ≤10 g/dL) with a restrictive strategy (hgb threshold ≤8 g/dL). The trial showed lower mortality with the liberal strategy. However, these findings require replication in a larger study.[9]
- Based on this and other studies, guidelines recommend a transfusion hgb threshold of <7 g/dL for most critically ill patients.[10]

Summary and Implications: For most critically ill patients, waiting to transfuse red cells until the hgb drops below 7.0 is at least as effective as, and likely preferable to, transfusing at a hgb less than 10.0. These findings may not apply to patients with chronic anemia, who were excluded from the trial. The results also may not apply to patients with active cardiac ischemia, who were poorly represented in the trial and had nonsignificantly worse outcomes with a transfusion threshold of 7.0.

CLINICAL CASE: RED CELL TRANSFUSION IN CRITICALLY ILL PATIENTS

Case History:

A 74-year-old woman with myelodysplastic syndrome is admitted to the general medicine service at your hospital with pneumonia. On review of systems, you note that she has suffered from increasing fatigue for the past 3 months. Her hgb on admission is 8.0 g/dL—which has decreased from 10.5 g/dL when it was last measured 4 months ago.

Based on the results of the TRICC trial, should you give this patient a red cell transfusion?

Suggested Answer:

The TRICC trial showed that, for most critically ill patients, waiting to transfuse red cells until the hgb drops below 7.0 g/dL is at least as effective as, and likely preferable to, transfusing at an hgb <10.0 g/dL. However, the patient in this vignette is not critically ill, and thus the results of TRICC should not be applied to her. This patient's fatigue likely results from anemia due to her myelodysplastic syndrome. Red cell transfusion would likely be appropriate for her.

References

1. Hébert PC et al. A multicenter, randomized, controlled clinical trial of transfusion requirements in critical care. *N Engl J Med.* 1999;340(6):409–417.
2. Hébert PC et al. Is a low transfusion threshold safe in critically ill patients with cardiovascular diseases? *Crit Care Med.* 2001;29(2):227.
3. Carless PA et al. Transfusion thresholds and other strategies for guiding allogeneic red blood cell transfusion. *Cochrane Database Syst Rev.* 2010;(10):CD002042.
4. Bracey AW et al. Lowering the hemoglobin threshold for transfusion in coronary artery bypass procedures: effect on patient outcome. *Transfusion.* 1999;39(10):1070.
5. Carson JL et al. Liberal or restrictive transfusion in high-risk patients after hip surgery. *N Engl J Med.* 2011;365(26):2453.
6. Robertson CS et al. Effect of erythropoietin and transfusion threshold on neurological recovery after traumatic brain injury: a randomized clinical trial. *JAMA.* 2014 Jul 2;312(1):36–47.
7. Lacroix J et al. Transfusion strategies for patients in pediatric intensive care units. *N Engl J Med.* 2007;356(16):1609–1619.
8. Villanueva C et al. Transfusion strategies for acute upper gastrointestinal bleeding. *N Engl J Med.* 2013;368(1):11–21.
9. Foss NB et al. The effects of liberal vs. restrictive transfusion thresholds on ambulation after hip fracture surgery. *Transfusion.* 2009;49(2):227.
10. Napolitano LM et al. Clinical practice guideline: red blood cell transfusion in adult trauma and critical care. *Crit Care Med.* 2009;37(12):3124.

38

Noninvasive Ventilation for Acute Exacerbations of Chronic Obstructive Pulmonary Disease

ADEL BOUEIZ

> Noninvasive ventilation in selected patients admitted for acute respiratory failure due to chronic obstructive pulmonary disease can obviate the need for intubation and thus reduce complications and mortality and shorten the hospital stay.
>
> —BROCHARD ET AL.[1]

Research Question: Is noninvasive mechanical ventilation effective among patients with acute exacerbations of chronic obstructive pulmonary disease (COPD)?[1]

Funding: Not reported.

Year Study Began: 1990

Year Study Published: 1995

Study Location: 5 hospitals in Europe (3 in France, 1 in Italy, 1 in Spain).

Who Was Studied: Adult patients with a known history of COPD admitted for an acute exacerbation of COPD with dyspnea of less than 2 weeks, respiratory acidosis, elevated bicarbonate, and two of the following three criteria:

- Respiratory rate >30
- Arterial oxygen <45 mm Hg
- Arterial pH <7.35

Who Was Excluded: Patients with a tracheostomy or endotracheal intubation prior to admission, those with a respiratory rate <12 or requiring endotracheal intubation on admission, and patients receiving sedative drugs in the last 12 hours. Additionally, patients with "central nervous system disorders unrelated to hypercapnic encephalopathy or hypoxemia," those with cardiac arrest within the previous 5 days, those with a facial deformity, and those unwilling to undergo endotracheal intubation were excluded.

How Many Patients: 85

Study Overview: See Figure 38.1 for a summary of the study's design.

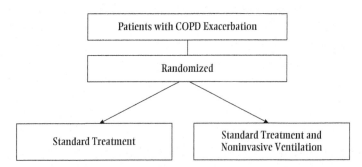

Figure 38.1 Summary of the Study Design.

Study Intervention: All patients were placed on oxygen by nasal cannula to target an oxygen saturation >90% with a maximum flow rate of 5 liters per minute. Patients also received subcutaneous heparin, antibiotics, bronchodilators, and management of electrolyte abnormalities (hereafter referred to as the standard treatment).

In addition to the standard treatment, patients in the noninvasive ventilation group received noninvasive positive-pressure ventilation (NPPV) for a minimum of 6 hours per day. The period of NPPV could be extended based on the clinical condition of the patient. NPPV was delivered via oronasal mask and provided pressure support triggered by the patient's inspiratory effort. Pressure support was initially set at 20 mm H_2O but could be adjusted to target an oxygen saturation >90%. If the patient stopped breathing while receiving NPPV, the mask delivered automatic pressure-controlled cycles.

Criteria for intubation included the presence of any of the major criteria listed below or at least two of the minor criteria (Table 38.1). If criteria for intubation were met by two minor criteria directly following NPPV withdrawal, NPPV could be reintroduced before proceeding to intubation.

Table 38.1 CRITERIA FOR INTUBATION

Major Criteria	Minor Criteria
Respiratory arrest	Respiratory rate >35 and higher than on admission
Respiratory pauses with loss of consciousness or gasping for air	Arterial pH <7.3 and lower than on admission
Psychomotor agitation requiring sedation	Partial pressure of oxygen <45 mm Hg despite oxygen therapy
Heart rate <50 with loss of alertness	An increase in encephalopathy score
Hemodynamic instability with systolic blood pressure <90 mm Hg	

Follow-Up: Until discharge from the hospital or death, whichever came first.

Endpoints: Primary outcome: Need for endotracheal intubation and mechanical ventilation. Secondary outcomes: Length of hospital stay, incidence of complications not present on admission (e.g., infections, myocardial infarction, or pulmonary embolism), duration of ventilatory assistance, and in-hospital mortality.

RESULTS

- Patients in both groups received similar treatment with antibiotics, bronchodilators, corticosteroids, and diuretics.
- Significantly fewer patients in the NPPV group required endotracheal intubation compared to patients in the standard-therapy group (Table 38.2).
- The length of hospital stay and the overall complication rate were higher in the standard-therapy group versus the NPPV group (Table 38.2).

- In-hospital mortality was lower in the NPPV group versus the standard-therapy group (Table 38.2); this difference was absent after adjusting for use of endotracheal intubation, which suggests that the benefits observed with noninvasive ventilation resulted from the lower number of patients requiring intubation.

Table 38.2 SUMMARY OF KEY FINDINGS

	Standard Treatment	Noninvasive Ventilation	*P* Value
Need for Endotracheal Intubation	74%	26%	<0.001
Length of Hospital Stay	35±33 days	23±17 days	0.02
Frequency of Complications Not Present on Admission	48%	16%	0.001
In-Hospital Mortality Rate	29%	9%	0.02

Criticisms and Limitations: Oxygen delivered by nasal prongs was limited to a flow rate of 5 liters per minute, which may have led to inadequate oxygenation and may have resulted in suboptimal medical management leading to the unusually high intubation rate (74%) observed in the standard-therapy group and exaggerating the apparent benefits of NPPV. The higher-than-expected intubation rate may also suggest that study patients were sicker than the typical patient with COPD, limiting the generalizability of the study results.

Other Relevant Studies and Information:

- A meta-analysis of 14 randomized controlled trials and 758 patients that compared standard therapy versus NPPV found that NPPV led to reductions in mortality (22% versus 11%), intubation rates (33% versus 16%), and treatment failure (42% versus 20%).[2]
- Another meta-analysis of 15 randomized controlled trials found the benefit of NPPV was only observed in patients with severe exacerbations of COPD defined as a baseline pH <7.3 or a mortality rate in the control group >10%.[3]
- The Global Initiative for Chronic Obstructive Lung Disease (GOLD) recommends initiation of NPPV in acute exacerbations of COPD in the presence of respiratory acidosis (pH <7.35 and/or arterial pressure of carbon dioxide >45 mm Hg) or severe dyspnea with signs of respiratory muscle fatigue.[4]

Summary and Implications: Among patients with acute exacerbations of COPD, NPPV reduced the need for endotracheal intubation, lowered complication rates and mortality, and shortened the hospital length of stay. GOLD now recommends NPPV for patients with severe COPD exacerbations.

CLINICAL CASE: MANAGEMENT OF COPD EXACERBATION

Case History:

A 69-year-old man presents with a 3-day history of progressive cough productive of purulent sputum and increasing dyspnea. He was diagnosed with COPD 2 years ago and has been maintained on as-needed bronchodilators. He smokes a pack of cigarettes per day. On physical examination, he is in moderate respiratory distress with a respiratory rate of 35, an oxygen saturation of 88% on room air, and bilateral expiratory wheezes. An arterial blood gas on room air reveals a pH of 7.30, $PaCO_2$ of 61 mm Hg, and a PaO_2 of 53 mm Hg. Which therapies would be most appropriate for this patient?

Suggested Answer:

This patient meets the definition of a severe exacerbation of COPD with increased dyspnea, sputum volume, and sputum purulence and should be medically managed with short-acting bronchodilators (β_2-agonists and anticholinergic agents), systemic corticosteroids, and antibiotics. In addition, given the presence of respiratory acidosis on admission, initiating NPPV is likely to reduce his risk for endotracheal intubation, complications, and mortality, and it could shorten his length of hospital stay.

References

1. Brochard L et al. Noninvasive ventilation for acute exacerbations of chronic obstructive pulmonary disease. *N Engl J Med*. 1995 Sep 28;333(13):817–822.
2. Ram FS, Picot J, Lightowler J, Wedzicha JA. Non-invasive positive pressure ventilation for treatment of respiratory failure due to exacerbations of chronic obstructive pulmonary disease. *Cochrane Database Syst Rev*. 2004;CD004104.
3. Keenan SP, Sinuff T, Cook DJ, Hill NS. Which patients with acute exacerbation of chronic obstructive pulmonary disease benefit from noninvasive positive-pressure ventilation? A systematic review of the literature. *Ann Intern Med*. 2003;138:861.
4. Global Initiative for Chronic Obstructive Lung Disease (GOLD). Global strategy for the diagnosis, management, and prevention of chronic obstructive pulmonary disease: revised 2013. www.goldcopd.org. Accessed December 9, 2013.

39

Low Tidal Volume Ventilation in Acute Respiratory Distress Syndrome/Acute Lung Injury

The ARDSNet Trial

KRISTOPHER SWIGER

> In patients with acute lung injury and the acute respiratory distress syndrome, mechanical ventilation with a lower tidal volume . . . results in decreased mortality and increases the number of days without ventilator use.
>
> —THE ARDS NETWORK INVESTIGATORS[1]

Research Question: Should patients with acute lung injury (ALI)/acute respiratory distress syndrome (ARDS) be managed with low tidal volume ventilation?[1]

Funding: The National Heart, Lung, and Blood Institute.

Year Study Began: 1996

Year Study Published: 2000

Study Location: 10 university centers in the United States.

Who Was Studied: Adults who were intubated and met the American-European Consensus Conference definition of ALI/ARDS,[2] defined as follows:

1. Ratio of partial pressure of arterial oxygen to fraction of inspired oxygen ≤300
2. Bilateral infiltrates on a chest x-ray consistent with pulmonary edema
3. No clinical evidence of left atrial hypertension

By the 2012 Berlin Classification, what was at the time of the study defined as ALI is now referred to as mild ARDS.

Who Was Excluded: Patients were excluded if it had been more than 36 hours since they met the inclusion criteria. In addition, the following groups were excluded: children, pregnant women, patients with serious comorbidities such as increased intracranial pressure or "neuromuscular disease that could impair spontaneous breathing," severe chronic respiratory disease, chronic liver disease, or other comorbidities that carried "an estimated 6-month mortality rate of more than 50 percent."

How Many Patients: 861

Study Overview: See Figure 39.1 for a summary of the study design.

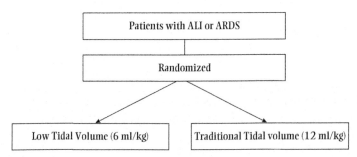

Figure 39.1 Summary of the Study Design.

Study Intervention: All patients received volume-assist-control ventilation. The traditional tidal volume group initially received a tidal volume of 12 mL per kilogram of predicted body weight, which "was subsequently reduced step-wise by 1 ml per kilogram of predicted body weight if necessary to maintain" a plateau pressure of 50 cm of water or less. Patients in the low tidal volume group initially received a tidal volume of 6 mL per kilogram, which "was subsequently reduced stepwise by 1 ml per kilogram of predicted body weight if necessary to maintain plateau pressure . . . of no more than 30 cm of water."

Follow-Up: 180 days.

Endpoints: Primary outcomes: Death before discharge and number of days without ventilator use from day 1 to 28. Secondary outcomes: Number of days without organ failure.

RESULTS

- The trial was stopped early when it became clear that the use of lower tidal volumes was beneficial (Table 39.1).
- Plateau pressures (which represent the pressure applied to small airways and alveoli during mechanical ventilation inspiration) were significantly lower in the group treated with lower tidal volumes.
- Positive end-expiratory pressure and fraction of inspired oxygen were significantly higher in the low tidal volume group on days 1 and 3, though the absolute differences were small and of questionable clinical significance. On day 7, these measures were higher in the traditional volume group.

Table 39.1 SUMMARY OF KEY FINDINGS

Outcome	Low Tidal Volume	Traditional Tidal Volume	P Value
Death before Discharge	31.0%	39.8%	0.007
Number of Ventilator-Free Days	12	10	0.007
Number of Days without Failure of Nonpulmonary Organs or Systems	15	11	0.006

Criticisms and Limitations: Some believe the trial used unconventionally high plateau pressures for the traditional tidal volume group, which may have been harmful and resulted in an overestimation of the benefit of low tidal volume ventilation. However, the majority of patients in the traditional volume group had plateau pressures <45 cm H_2O.

Other Relevant Studies and Information:

- Two meta-analyses involving ten randomized trials are concordant with the ARDSNet trial results.[3,4]
- The 2012 Surviving Sepsis Campaign Guidelines recommend a target tidal volume of 6 mL/kg predicted body weight for mechanical ventilation in patients with sepsis-induced ARDS.[5]

Summary and Implications: In patients with ALI or ARDS, mechanical ventilation with a lower tidal volume decreases in-hospital mortality and increases the number of days alive without ventilator dependence or organ failure. This study helped confirm the concept that gentler ventilation by limiting pressure on the small airways and alveoli is the optimal strategy for managing patients with ARDS.

CLINICAL CASE: LOW TIDAL VOLUME VENTILATION

Case History:
A 79-year-old woman is hospitalized for a hip fracture. On her fifth day of hospitalization she becomes progressively hypoxemic, is diagnosed with hospital-acquired pneumonia, and requires mechanical ventilation for hypoxic respiratory failure. A chest x-ray reveals bilateral, diffuse alveolar infiltrates. Her partial pressure of oxygen in an arterial blood (PaO2) is 100 on a fraction of inspired oxygen (FiO2) of 80%.

Based on the results by the ARDS Network Investigators, how should this patient be treated?

Suggested Answer:
The study in question showed that low tidal volume ventilation decreases mortality in the hospital and reduces the number of days alive and on mechanical ventilation. This is driven by a decrease in plateau pressure and lung distension.

The patient in question is typical of those at risk of ARDS and those studied by the ARDS Network Investigators. The recommended ventilation strategy for patients with ARDS is volume-assist-control with an initial tidal volume of 8 mL/kilogram of predicted body weight. This should be further reduced down to 6 mL/kg of predicted body weight (as demonstrated by the ARDS Network Investigators) while maintaining plateau pressure less than 30 cm H_2O and oxygenation and ventilation as close to normal as possible.

References

1. The ARDS Network. Ventilation with lower tidal volumes as compared with traditional tidal volumes for ALI and ARDS. *N Engl J Med.* 2000;342:1301–1308.

2. Bernard GR et al. The American-European Consensus Conference on ARDS: definitions, mechanics, relevant outcomes and clinical trial coordination. *Am J Respir Crit Care Med.* 1994;149:818–824.

3. Petrucci N, Iacovelli W. Ventilation with lower tidal volumes versus traditional tidal volumes in adults for acute lung injury and acute respiratory distress syndrome. *Cochrane Database Syst Rev.* 2004;2:CD003844. doi: 10.1002/14651858. CD003844.pub2.

4. Putensen C et al. Meta-analysis: ventilation strategies and outcomes of the acute respiratory distress syndrome and acute lung injury. *Annals Intern Med.* 2009 Oct;151(8):566–576.

5. Dellinger RP et al. Surviving sepsis campaign: international guidelines for management of severe sepsis and septic shock, 2012. *Intensive Care Med.* 2013;39(2):165–228. doi:10.1007/s00134-012-2769-8.

40

Comparison of Routine versus On-Demand Chest Radiographs in Mechanically Ventilated Adults in the Intensive Care Unit

ADEL BOUEIZ

Results from our study show a substantial reduction in use of chest radiographs with the on-demand strategy . . . [with] similar . . . duration of mechanical ventilation and stay in the intensive care unit, and mortality.

—HEJBLUM ET AL.[1]

Research Question: Are daily, routine chest radiographs necessary in mechanically ventilated adults versus an as-needed strategy?[1]

Funding: Assistance Publique-Hôpitaux de Paris, a public hospital system serving Paris and its suburbs.

Year Study Began: 2006

Year Study Published: 2009

Study Location: 21 intensive care units (ICUs; 13 medical, 2 surgical, and 6 mixed) in Paris, France (17 located at university hospitals).

Who Was Studied: Adult patients in ICUs receiving mechanical ventilation.

Who Was Excluded: Patients on mechanical ventilation for fewer than 2 days were enrolled in the protocol but were not included in the analysis.

How Many Patients: 849

Study Overview: See Figure 40.1 for a summary of the study design.

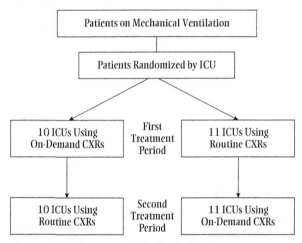

Figure 40.1 Summary of the Study Design.

Study Intervention: All patients in both groups received an initial chest radiograph after intubation.

In the routine, daily chest x-ray group, all mechanically ventilated patients received a chest x-ray at the time of morning rounds regardless of clinical condition. Patients also received any other chest radiographs deemed necessary throughout the day.

In the on-demand group, patients received chest x-rays only when warranted by clinical findings.

Each ICU followed the assigned protocol until 20 patients had been enrolled and completed their follow-up (discharge from the ICU or 30 days on mechanical ventilation, whichever came first). This was followed by a one-week washout period, after which each ICU switched to the other strategy (i.e., ICUs using an on-demand approach switched to a routine, daily chest x-ray approach and vice versa).

Follow-Up: 30 days on mechanical ventilation or discharge from ICU, whichever occurred first.

Endpoints: Primary outcome: Mean number of chest x-rays per patient-day of mechanical ventilation (excluding initial chest x-ray following intubation). Secondary outcomes: Days of mechanical ventilation, length of ICU stay, and ICU mortality.

RESULTS

- Patients randomized to the on-demand chest radiography strategy had a 32% reduction in the mean number of chest x-rays per patient-day of mechanical ventilation compared to those allocated to the routine strategy (Table 40.1).
- Despite fewer chest x-rays performed using the on-demand strategy, there were no differences in the number of x-rays with clinically meaningful findings requiring intervention between the groups (Table 40.1).
- The duration of mechanical ventilation, length of ICU stay, and ICU mortality were similar between the groups (Table 40.1).

Table 40.1 SUMMARY OF KEY FINDINGS

	On-Demand	Routine	*P* Value
Mean Number of Chest X-Rays per Patient-Day of Mechanical Ventilation	0.75	1.09	<0.001
Number of Chest X-Rays Requiring Further Diagnostic or Therapeutic Intervention	729	728	0.77
Mean Duration of Mechanical Ventilation (Days)	9.9	9.8	0.90
Mean Length of ICU Stay (Days)	13.21	13.96	0.28
ICU Mortality	32%	31%	nonsignificant[a]

[a] Actual *P* value not reported.

Criticisms and Limitations: Though the study detected a significant reduction in the number of chest radiographs ordered per patient-day of mechanical ventilation, it was not powered to detect clinically important differences in morbidity and mortality. Additionally, the study authors did not provide criteria for when to order chest x-rays on an as-needed basis. Finally, the study did not indicate how long it is safe for a mechanically ventilated patient to go without receiving a chest x-ray.

Other Relevant Studies and Information:

- A meta-analysis of eight trials comparing routine versus on-demand chest radiography among 7,078 ICU patients found that the two strategies resulted in similar mortality, hospital and ICU length of stay, and days of mechanical ventilation.[2]
- The Society for Critical Care Medicine guidelines for management of patients with acute respiratory failure on mechanical ventilation recommends an initial chest radiograph and further radiographs only as clinically indicated.[3]
- The American College of Radiology recommends chest radiographs only as indicated by clinical conditions among patients with acute cardiopulmonary problems.[4]

Summary and Implications: Critically ill, mechanically ventilated patients who receive chest x-rays only as needed receive fewer total x-rays and have similar outcomes as patients who receive daily chest x-rays. These results have been replicated in multiple studies involving a wide variety of ICU patients. Based on these findings, guidelines recommend chest radiography for mechanically ventilated patients only as needed.

CLINICAL CASE: CHEST X-RAYS IN THE ICU

Case History:
A 60-year-old woman with urosepsis and multiple organ dysfunction is admitted to the ICU and intubated and mechanically ventilated for worsening hypoxic respiratory failure. Based on the results of this trial, how should chest radiography be used to follow this patient's progress in the ICU?

Suggested Answer:
Ordering chest radiography in response to specific clinical circumstances (i.e., on-demand) as opposed to routine, daily chest radiography is likely to result in fewer chest x-rays ordered per day of mechanical ventilation without adversely impacting her outcome. Thus, the on-demand approach is preferable.

References

1. Hejblum G et al. Comparison of routine and on-demand prescription of chest radiographs in mechanically ventilated adults: a multicentre, cluster-randomised, two-period crossover study. *Lancet.* 2009;374(9702):1687–1693.
2. Oba Y, Zaza T. Abandoning daily routine chest radiography in the intensive care unit: meta-analysis. *Radiology.* 2010;255(2):386–395.
3. Task Force on Guidelines, Society of Critical Care Medicine. Guidelines for standard of care for patients with acute respiratory failure on mechanical ventilator support. *Crit Care Med.* 1991;19:275–278.
4. Expert Panel on Thoracic Imaging. ACR appropriateness criteria routine chest radiographs in intensive care unit patients. *J Am Coll Radiol.* 2013;10(3):170–174.

41

Early Goal-Directed Therapy in Sepsis

MICHAEL E. HOCHMAN

[Immediate recognition and management] of severe sepsis and septic shock . . . has significant short-term and long-term benefits.

—RIVERS ET AL.[1]

Research Question: Does immediate recognition and management of sepsis improve outcomes?[1]

Funding: Henry Ford Health Systems Fund for Research and a Weatherby Healthcare Resuscitation Fellowship.

Year Study Began: 1997

Year Study Published: 2001

Study Location: The Henry Ford Hospital in Detroit, Michigan.

Who Was Studied: Adults presenting to the emergency room with severe sepsis or septic shock. To qualify, patients needed to have a suspected infection and at least two of four criteria for a systemic inflammatory response syndrome (SIRS) as well as a systolic blood pressure ≤90 mm Hg. Alternatively, they could have a suspected infection, at least two SIRS criteria, and a lactate ≥4.0 mm/L (Table 41.1).

Table 41.1 SIRS Criteria

Temperature	≤36°C (96.8°F) or ≥38°C (100.4°F)
Heart Rate	≥90
Respiratory Rate	≥20 or $PaCO_2$ <32 mm Hg
White Cell Count	≥12,000 or ≤4,000 or ≥10% bands

Who Was Excluded: Patients who were pregnant, as well as those with several acute conditions including stroke, acute coronary syndrome, acute pulmonary edema, status asthmaticus, or gastrointestinal bleeding. In addition, patients with a contraindication to central venous catheterization were excluded.

How Many Patients: 263

Study Overview: See Figure 41.1 for a summary of the trial's design.

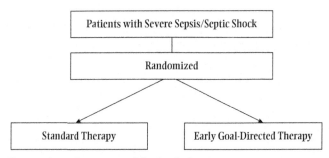

Figure 41.1 Summary of the Study Design.

Study Intervention: Patients in the standard-therapy group received immediate critical care consultation and were admitted to the intensive care unit (ICU) as quickly as possible. Subsequent management was at the discretion of the critical care team, which was given a protocol advocating the following hemodynamic goals:

- 500-mL boluses of crystalloid should be given every 30 minutes as needed to achieve a central venous pressure (CVP) of 8–12 mm Hg.
- Vasopressors should be used as needed to maintain a mean arterial pressure (MAP) ≥65 mm Hg.
- Urine output goal ≥0.5 mL/kg/h.

Patients in the early goal-directed therapy group were managed according to a similar protocol. However, they also received central venous oxygen saturation ($ScvO_2$) monitoring from a specialized central line catheter:

- If the $ScvO_2$ was <70%, red cells were transfused to achieve a hematocrit ≥30%.
- If the transfusion was ineffective, dobutamine was given as tolerated.

In addition, and perhaps most importantly, patients in the early goal-directed therapy group received 6 hours of aggressive treatment *immediately* upon presentation to the emergency room.

Follow-Up: 60 days.

Endpoints: Primary outcome: In-hospital mortality.

RESULTS

- During the first 6 hours, patients in the early goal-directed therapy group received more fluid, more blood transfusions, and more inotropic support than did patients in the standard-therapy group.
- During the first 6 hours, patients in the early goal-directed group had higher average MAPs, and a higher average $ScvO_2$; in addition, a higher proportion achieved the combined goals for CVP, MAP, and urine output.
- During the period from 7 to 72 hours, patients in the early goal-directed therapy group had better hemodynamic parameters and required less fluid, red cell transfusions, vasopressors, and mechanical ventilation.
- Mortality was lower in the early goal-directed therapy group (see Table 41.2).

Table 41.2 SUMMARY OF KEY FINDINGS

Outcome	Standard-Therapy Group	Early Goal-Directed Therapy Group	P Value
Hospital Length of Stay[a]	18.4 days	14.6 days	0.04
60-Day Mortality	56.9%	44.3%	0.03
In-Hospital Mortality	46.5%	30.5%	0.009

[a] Among patients who survived to hospital discharge.

Criticisms and Limitations: The early goal-directed protocol involved several interventions, not all of which have subsequently proven to be necessary to achieve optimal outcomes for patients with sepsis. In particular, recent studies noted below have suggested that aggressive red cell transfusions and dobuta-mine administration based on $ScvO_2$ measurements are likely not necessary.

Other Relevant Studies and Information:

- A trial comparing hemodynamic monitoring with $ScvO_2$ measurements versus lactate clearance in patients with sepsis suggested that the two forms of monitoring are equivalent.[2]
- A trial comparing early goal-directed therapy, "protocol-based standard therapy that did not require the placement of a central venous catheter, administration of inotropes, or blood transfusions," and usual care found no differences in outcomes among the treatment strategies.[3] This follow-up study suggests that invasive monitoring and aggressive targeting of hemodynamic parameters are likely not necessary, but rather the focus of managing sepsis should be on "early recognition . . . early administration of antibiotics, early adequate volume resuscitation, and clinical assessment of the adequacy of circulation."[4] In other words, this study refines our understanding by highlighting that immediate recognition and management of sepsis— rather than aggressive targeting of hemodynamic parameters—are what drive optimal sepsis outcomes.
- Another subsequent trial also failed to demonstrate a benefit of early goal-directed therapy vs. standard therapy involving immediate antibiotics and fluids but without specific hemodynamic targets.[5]

Summary and Implications: Patients with severe sepsis or septic shock who were managed immediately with aggressive therapy had better outcomes than those managed less aggressively. Follow-up studies have suggested that much of the benefit of early aggressive therapy likely result not from aggressive hemo-dynamic monitoring and targeting but rather from early recognition of sepsis with immediate antibiotic administration and volume resuscitation and close clinical monitoring. When patients with sepsis are recognized, antibiotics, fluid resuscitation, and close clinical monitoring should begin immediately.

CLINICAL CASE: EARLY GOAL-DIRECTED THERAPY

Case History:
A 48-year-old previously healthy man presents, reporting that he "feels mis-erable." Over the past day, he has had a cough with thick green sputum as well as subjective fevers and fatigue. The symptoms worsened 2 hours prior to

presentation, and he now has rigors, increasing fatigue, and mild to moderate dyspnea. On exam, his temperature is 39°C (102.2°F), his heart rate is 126, his respiratory rate is 24, and his blood pressure is 86 mm Hg/60 mm Hg. His labs are notable for a white blood cell count of 18,000 with 40% bands and a lactate of 3.0 mm/L. His chest X-ray shows a right middle lobe consolidation.

After reading this trial about early goal-directed therapy, and considering key follow-up studies, how would you treat this patient upon presentation to the emergency room?

Suggested Answer:

This patient fulfills the criteria for severe sepsis. He should be treated immediately with antibiotics and fluid resuscitation. Based on recent studies, it is likely unnecessary to perform invasive hemodynamic monitoring with $ScvO_2$ measurements. However, he should be monitored very closely with clinical assessments and lactate measurements as needed. Fluids and vasopressors should be used to optimize tissue perfusion based on these assessments.

References

1. Rivers E et al. Early goal-directed therapy in the treatment of severe sepsis and septic shock. *N Engl J Med.* 2001;345(19):1368–1377.
2. Jones AE et al. Lactate clearance vs. central venous oxygen saturation as goals of early sepsis therapy: a randomized clinical trial. *JAMA.* 2010;303(8):739–746.
3. The ProCESS Investigators. A randomized trial of protocol-based care for early septic shock. *N Engl J Med.* 2014 May 1;370(18):1683–1693.
4. Lilly CM. The ProCESS trial—a new era of sepsis management. *N Engl J Med.* 2014 May 1;370(18):1750–1751.
5. ARISE Investigators; ANZICS Clinical Trials Group, Peake SL, Delaney A, Bailey M, Bellomo R, Cameron PA, Cooper DJ, Higgins AM, Holdgate A, Howe BD, Webb SA, Williams P. Goal-directed resuscitation for patients with early septic shock. *N Engl J Med.* 2014 Oct 16;371(16):1496–506.

Dopamine versus Norepinephrine in the Treatment of Shock

ADEL BOUEIZ

Among patients with all types of shock, norepinephrine and dopamine compare similarly with respect to 28-day mortality, but dopamine is associated with an increased risk of arrhythmias. Norepinephrine may have a mortality benefit over dopamine in a subset of patients with cardiogenic shock.

—De Backer et al.[1]

Research Question: Is dopamine or norepinephrine a better first-line vasopressor in patients with shock?[1]

Funding: European Critical Care Research Network.

Year Study Began: 2003

Year Study Published: 2010

Study Location: Eight centers in Belgium, Austria, and Spain.

Who Was Studied: Patients over age 18 with shock, defined as a mean arterial pressure (MAP) <70 mm Hg or systolic blood pressure <100 mm Hg despite adequate fluid resuscitation (at least 1 L crystalloid or 500 cc colloids), with signs of "tissue hypoperfusion" such as altered mental status, "mottled skin," decreased urine output, or increased serum lactate.

Who Was Excluded: Patients who received a vasopressor for at least 4 hours prior to enrollment, had a "serious arrhythmia" (e.g., rapid atrial fibrillation >160 beats/min or ventricular tachycardia), or had been diagnosed with brain death.

How Many Patients: 1,679

Study Overview: See Figure 42.1 for a summary of the study's design.

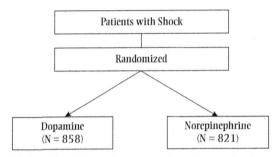

Figure 42.1 Summary of the Study Design.

Study Intervention: Patients were initiated on a weight-based dose of dopamine or norepinephrine that was titrated at the discretion of the treating physicians with maximum doses not to exceed 20 mcg/kg/min for dopamine and 0.19 mcg/kg/min for norepinephrine. Any vasopressor the patient was on prior to randomization was discontinued and replaced by the study drug as soon as possible. If the patient remained hypotensive despite maximal doses of the study drug, norepinephrine was initiated.

Follow-Up: 28 days.

Endpoints: Primary outcome: All-cause mortality at 28 days. Secondary outcomes: Mortality in the intensive care unit (ICU) or hospital; mortality at 6 and 12 months; number of days without need for vasopressor support; and the occurrence of adverse events.

RESULTS

- There were no differences in mortality between the two groups (Table 42.1).

- Patients in the norepinephrine group required less vasopressor support than those in the dopamine group.
- More patients in the dopamine group than the norepinephrine group experienced arrhythmias (24.1% versus 12.4%, $P < 0.001$).
- In a predefined subgroup analysis, among patients with cardiogenic shock, 28-day mortality was lower in patients in the norepinephrine group ($P = 0.03$).

Table 42.1 SUMMARY OF KEY FINDINGS

Time Period	Dopamine	Norepinephrine	P Value
Mortality			
In ICU	50.2%	45.9%	0.07
During Hospitalization	59.4%	56.6%	0.24
At 28 Days	52.5%	48.5%	0.10
At 6 Months	63.8%	62.9%	0.71
At 12 Months	65.9%	63.0%	0.34

Criticisms and Limitations: The study authors included patients who were hypotensive despite receiving 1 L of crystalloids or 0.5 L of colloids. However, this is a lenient definition of fluid-resistant shock. The authors have also been criticized for not clearly stating the definition for the resolution of shock.

Other Relevant Studies:

- This study was prompted by an observational study showing that patients with shock who were treated with dopamine had higher ICU (43% versus 36%, $P = 0.02$) and hospital (50% versus 42%, $P = 0.01$) mortality than those treated with norepinephrine.[2]
- A meta-analysis of six randomized trials involving 1,408 patients with septic shock showed that patients who received dopamine had higher 28-day mortality than patients who received norepinephrine (54% versus 49%, RR 1.12, 95% confidence interval 1.01–1.20).[3]
- The Society of Critical Care Medicine's 2012 guidelines on sepsis recommend norepinephrine as the first-line vasopressor for sepsis.[4]

Summary and Implications: In patients with shock, there was no significant difference in the mortality rates between patients treated with norepinephrine compared to dopamine. However, arrhythmias were less common in the norepinephrine group, and mortality was lower among a subgroup of patients with cardiogenic shock. Overall, results from this study and others suggest that norepinephrine is superior to dopamine for the management of shock, and guidelines now recommend norepinephrine as the first-line vasopressor agent.

CLINICAL CASE: FIRST-LINE VASOPRESSOR IN SEPTIC SHOCK

Case History:

A 49-year-old woman with acute myelogenous leukemia is in the ICU with neutropenia, ascending cholangitis, and septic shock. Upon arrival to the emergency room, she was resuscitated with intravenous crystalloid, started on broad-spectrum antibiotics, and intubated for shock. Vital signs in the ICU were a temperature of 37.2°C (99.0°F), heart rate of 110, a blood pressure of 80/40, and a respiratory rate of 20. The patient has been oliguric. Based on the results of this study, what is the appropriate next step in the management of this patient?

Suggested Answer:

It is important, first, to make sure that the patient is adequately resuscitated with fluids before administering vasopressors. If a vasopressor is indicated, norepinephrine is the recommended first-line agent.

References

1. De Backer D et al. Comparison of dopamine and norepinephrine in the treatment of shock. *N Engl J Med*. 2010 Mar 4;362(9):779–789.
2. Sakr Y et al. Does dopamine administration in shock influence outcomes? Results of the Sepsis Occurrence in Acutely Ill Patients (SOAP) Study. *Crit Care Med*. 2006 Mar;34(3):589–597.
3. De Backer D, Aldecoa C, Njimi H, Vincent JL. Dopamine versus norepinephrine in the treatment of septic shock: a meta-analysis. *Crit Care Med*. 2012;40(3):725–730.
4. Surviving Sepsis Campaign Guidelines Committee, Society of Critical Care Medicine. Surviving sepsis campaign: international guidelines for management of severe sepsis and septic shock, 2012. *Crit Care Med*. 2013;41(2):580–637.

Daily Interruption of Sedative Infusions in Critically Ill Patients Undergoing Mechanical Ventilation

LAALITHA SURAPANENI

> Daily interruption . . . of sedative drugs . . . decreases the duration of mechanical ventilation, the length of stay in the intensive care unit, and the doses of benzodiazepines used.
>
> —KRESS ET AL.[1]

Research Question: Does daily interruption of sedative infusions in critically ill patients receiving mechanical ventilation decrease the duration of mechanical ventilation and the duration of stay in the intensive care unit (ICU)?[1]

Funding: Not reported.

Year Study Began: Not reported

Year Study Published: 2000

Study Location: 1 medical ICU in the United States.

Who Was Studied: Critically ill patients on mechanical ventilation and requiring continuous sedative infusions.

Who Was Excluded: Patients admitted from an outside facility where they had already received sedative medications, those who were pregnant, and patients who had been resuscitated from a cardiac arrest. Patients who died or were extubated within 48 hours of enrollment were also excluded.

How Many Patients: 128

Study Overview: See Figure 43.1 for a summary of the study's design.

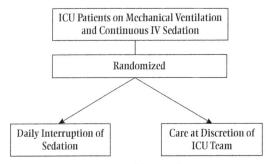

Figure 43.1 Summary of the Study Design.

Study Intervention: Patients in both groups were randomized to receive either midazolam or propofol, and all patients received morphine for analgesia. Forty-eight hours following enrollment, patients in the intervention group were removed from continuous sedative infusion once per day by a study physician until they were awake and able to follow commands or showed signs of being uncomfortable or agitated. Patients were classified as "awake" if they could complete at least three of the following: open their eyes in response to a voice; follow an examiner with their eyes; squeeze hands upon prompting; and stick out tongue upon prompting. Subsequently, the sedative infusion was resumed at half the previous dose, if necessary. In both the intervention and control groups, all other medical decisions, including decisions about when to extubate patients, were left to the discretion of the treating physicians.

Follow-Up: Until hospital discharge or death, whichever came first.

Endpoints: Primary outcomes: Duration of mechanical ventilation, length of ICU stay, and length of hospital stay. Secondary outcomes: Percentage of days the patient was awake at any point during the day, total doses of midazolam or propofol and morphine administered, and adverse events resulting from patient agitation such as the removal of the endotracheal tube by the patient.

RESULTS

- Patients undergoing daily interruption of sedative infusion had fewer days of mechanical ventilation and shorter stays in the ICU than patients in the control group and were awake a greater percentage of days compared to the control group (Table 43.1).
- Among patients sedated with midazolam, the total dose of midazolam and morphine was lower in the intervention versus control group ($P = 0.05$ and $P = 0.009$, respectively); there was no significant difference in the dose of propofol between the two groups.
- The control group required more diagnostic tests (CT scans, MRIs, and lumbar punctures) to assess changes in mental status compared to the intervention group (16 versus 6 tests, $P = 0.02$).
- There were no significant differences in adverse events or mortality rates between the groups.

Table 43.1 SUMMARY OF KEY FINDINGS

Variable	Intervention Group	Control Group	P Value
Duration of Mechanical Ventilation (Days)	4.9 days	7.3 days	0.004
Length of Stay in ICU	6.4 days	9.9 days	0.02
Length of Hospital Stay	13.3 days	16.9 days	0.19
Percentage of Days Awake	85.5%	9.0%	<0.001

Criticisms and Limitations: Some have argued that the benefit noted in the intervention group may be related to oversedation in the control group as opposed to the sedation interruption in the intervention group. In addition, the study was conducted among medical ICU patients and may not be generalizable to patients in the neurological or surgical ICU. Lastly, the study was not sufficiently powered to detect differences in complications such as self-extubation and there was no assessment of cardiovascular endpoints.

Other Relevant Studies and Information:

- A study of 336 patients showed that daily sedation interruption resulted in lower one-year mortality, increased ventilator-free days, fewer days in the ICU, decreased hospital stay, and less short-term cognitive impairment than did conventional sedation management.[2]
- A trial of 430 patients randomized to protocol-driven sedative infusions with or without daily interruptions of sedative infusions

found no difference between the two groups. These findings suggest
that effective sedation-weaning protocols may be as beneficial as a
daily sedation interruption.[3]

- The Society of Critical Care Medicine guidelines recommend
daily sedation interruptions or targeting light levels of sedation in
mechanically ventilated, adult ICU patients.[4]

Summary and Implications: This was the first trial to demonstrate that daily
sedation interruption for mechanically ventilated medical ICU patients is a
safe, effective, and cost-conscious strategy for weaning patients from continuous IV sedation. Subsequent studies suggest that protocol-driven sedation
weaning may also be an effective strategy for weaning sedation. Clinical guidelines currently recommend daily complete or near-complete sedation interruptions for mechanically ventilated adult ICU patients.

CLINICAL CASE: SEDATION IN CRITICALLY ILL PATIENTS

Case History:

A 58-year-old man is admitted to the ICU and intubated for respiratory failure secondary to pneumonia. Etomidate was used to facilitate the intubation,
but soon after the effects of etomidate wore off, the patient was awake and
agitated, trying to pull out lines and tubes. Midazolam is started for sedation
and morphine for analgesia. Two days following sedation and intubation, the
patient has a score of 6 on the Ramsey sedation scale (an ICU sedation-grad-
ing scale with 6 indicative of deep sedation). Based on the results of this study,
how should this patient's sedation be managed?

Suggested Answer:

The Kress study demonstrated that daily interruption of sedation in critically
ill, ventilated patients decreases the duration of mechanical ventilation, time
in the ICU, and need for neurodiagnostic testing to evaluate for changes in
mental status.

Based on the results of the study, this patient's sedation (midazolam) and
analgesia (morphine) should be interrupted once a day until the patient is
awake and able to follow commands. Once fully awake, the physician taking
care of the patient should assess and determine the need for restarting the
continuous infusion of sedation.

> If at any point the patient is agitated or uncomfortable, the sedation should be resumed. After 24 hours, the patient should be given another sedation interruption and reassessed.

References

1. Kress JP, Pohlman AS, O'Connor MF, Hall JB. Daily interruption of sedative infusions in critically ill patients undergoing mechanical ventilation. *N Engl J Med.* 2000;342:1471.
2. Girard TD et al. Efficacy and safety of a paired sedation and ventilator weaning protocol for mechanically ventilated patients in intensive care (Awakening and Breathing Controlled trial): a randomised controlled trial. *Lancet.* 2008;371:126.
3. Mehta S et al. Daily sedation interruption in mechanically ventilated critically ill patients cared for with a sedation protocol: a randomized controlled trial. *JAMA.* 2012;308:1985.
4. Barr J et al. Clinical practice guidelines for the management of pain, agitation, and delirium in adult patients in the intensive care unit. *Crit Care Med.* 2013;41(1):263–306.

A Comparison of Four Methods of Weaning Patients from Mechanical Ventilation

LAALITHA SURAPANENI

A once-daily trial of spontaneous breathing led to extubation about three times more quickly than intermittent mandatory ventilation and about twice as quickly as pressure-support ventilation.

—ESTEBAN ET AL.[1]

Research Question: What is the best method for weaning mechanical ventilation in patients with an initial unsuccessful spontaneous breathing trial?[1]

Funding: Veterans Affairs Research Service.

Year Study Began: 1992

Year Study Published: 1995

Study Location: 14 medical-surgical intensive care units (ICUs) in Spain.

Who Was Studied: Patients on mechanical ventilation for more than 24 hours with "improvement in or resolution of the underlying cause of acute respiratory failure" and a ratio of arterial oxygen to fraction of inspired oxygen >200 with a positive end-expiratory pressure <5 cm H_2O. All patients randomized had been unsuccessfully extubated with a 2-hour spontaneous breathing trial.

Who Was Excluded: Patients with a hemoglobin less than 10 g/dL or a core temperature ≥38°C (100.4°F) as well as those with a continued need for sedation or vasoactive drugs or a tracheostomy.

How Many Patients: 130

Study Overview: See Figure 44.1 for a summary of the study's design.

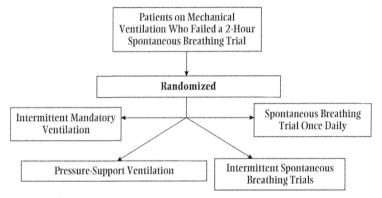

Figure 44.1 Summary of the Study Design.

Study Intervention: Patients who failed a 2-hour spontaneous breathing trial were termed "difficult to wean" and were then randomized to one of four weaning strategies:

1. Intermittent mandatory ventilation: Ventilation set at half of the initial respiratory rate with reductions in the rate at least two times per day as tolerated. Patients were extubated if they tolerated a respiratory rate of five breaths per minute for 2 hours.
2. Pressure-support ventilation: Pressure-support ventilation starting at 18 cm H_2O and reduced at least two times per day as tolerated. Patients were extubated if they tolerated pressure-support ventilation at a setting of 5 cm H_2O for 2 hours.
3. Intermittent trials of spontaneous breathing: Trials of spontaneous breathing were attempted at least twice daily, with mechanical ventilation between trials. The length of these trials was gradually increased and patients were extubated if they tolerated a trial for 2 hours.
4. Once-daily trial of spontaneous breathing: Once-daily trials of spontaneous breathing with mechanical ventilation between trials. Again, patients were extubated if they tolerated a trial for 2 hours.

Follow-Up: 48 hours following attempted extubation or 14 days from the time of enrollment if extubation was not achieved.

Endpoints: Median duration of weaning prior to successful extubation and rate of successful weaning defined as extubation within 14 days without need for reintubation.

RESULTS

- Of 546 patients eligible for enrollment in the trial, 416 (76%) were successfully extubated following the initial 2-hour spontaneous breathing trial and were not randomized.
- The rate of successful weaning was higher with a daily spontaneous breathing trial than with intermittent mandatory ventilation (rate ratio 2.83, $P < 0.006$) or pressure-support ventilation (rate ratio 2.05, $P < 0.04$); rate of successful extubation was similar between once-daily and intermittent spontaneous breathing trials (Table 44.1).
- The duration of weaning prior to successful extubation was shortest in the daily and intermittent spontaneous breathing trial groups (Table 44.1).

Table 44.1 SUMMARY OF KEY FINDINGS

Outcome	Intermittent Mandatory Ventilation	Pressure-Support Ventilation	Intermittent Spontaneous Breathing Trials	Once-Daily Spontaneous Breathing Trials
Median Duration of Weaning	5 days	4 days	3 days	3 days
Successful Weaning	69%	62%	82%	71%
Continued Mechanical Ventilation at 14 Days	17%	11%	3%	3%

Criticisms and Limitations: This study did not consider endpoints such as all-cause mortality, hospital-stay duration, and other important clinical outcomes. In addition, despite the wide representation of patient population, the sample size was small and patients were only followed for 14 days.

Other Relevant Studies and Information:

- A trial of 300 patients assigned to weaning from mechanical ventilation using spontaneous breathing trials versus weaning methods at the discretion of the treating physician showed a shorter period of attempted weaning, fewer complications associated with respiratory failure, as well as a reduction in the total cost of care with spontaneous breathing trials compared to other weaning methods.[2]

Summary and Implications: Among patients who were difficult to wean from mechanical ventilation, once-daily and intermittent trials of spontaneous breathing led to a higher rate of successful extubation with a shorter duration of weaning than did other weaning methods. There were no significant differences in weaning success rates between once-daily and intermittent spontaneous breathing trials. However, the once-daily method is simpler. It is notable that 76% of patients eligible for this trial were extubated with a single spontaneous breathing trial and did not require additional weaning techniques.

CLINICAL CASE: MODE OF WEANING FROM MECHANICAL VENTILATION

Case History:

A 65-year-old man is intubated for respiratory distress with a diagnosis of aspiration pneumonia and is treated with antibiotics for 8 days. He is now awake, following commands, and has an oxygen saturation of 99% on a fraction of inspired oxygen of 30% and no positive end-expiratory pressure. His respiratory rate is 22/min. A trial of spontaneous breathing is attempted, but within 20 minutes the patient develops respiratory distress and his oxygen saturation drops to 85%. The patient is placed back on mechanical ventilation.

Based on the results of the trial, what mode of mechanical ventilation weaning should be used for this patient?

Suggested Answer:

This study showed that weaning patients from mechanical ventilation with spontaneous breathing trials is superior to weaning using intermittent mandatory ventilation or pressure-supported ventilation in patients who fail an initial trial of spontaneous breathing. Spontaneous breathing trials have a higher probability of success, and they result in a shorter duration of mechanical ventilation. Once-daily spontaneous breathing trials appear to be as effective as intermittent breathing trials, but they provide a simpler protocol for weaning.

The patient in this vignette is similar to those included in the trial. He should thus be weaned using a spontaneous breathing trial. A once-daily trial would be sufficient.

References

1. Esteban A et al. A comparison of four methods of weaning patients from mechanical ventilation. Spanish Lung Failure Collaborative Group. *N Engl J Med.* 1995;332:345.
2. Ely EW et al. Effect on the duration of mechanical ventilation of identifying patients capable of breathing spontaneously. *N Engl J Med.* 1996;335:1864.

Geriatrics and Palliative Care

45

Behavioral versus Pharmacological Treatment for Insomnia in the Elderly

MICHAEL E. HOCHMAN

[These] findings indicate that behavioral and pharmacological therapies, alone or in combination, are effective in short-term management
of late-life insomnia . . . Follow-up results showed that behavior therapy
yielded the most durable improvements.

—MORIN ET AL.[1]

Research Question: Which is better for treating insomnia in the elderly: cog-
nitive-behavioral therapy (CBT), medications, or a combination of the two?[1]

Funding: The National Institute of Mental Health.

Year Study Began: The mid-1990s

Year Study Published: 1999

Study Location: An academic medical center in Virginia.

Who Was Studied: Adults ≥55 with either sleep-onset insomnia or
sleep-maintenance insomnia for at least 6 months. Sleep-onset insomnia was
defined as latency of sleep onset for more than 30 minutes at least three nights
a week, while sleep-maintenance insomnia was defined as waking after falling

asleep for more than 30 minutes at least three nights a week. To be eligible, patients also were required to have daytime symptoms such as fatigue.

Study patients were recruited through letters to physicians and newspaper advertisements. Volunteers underwent an intensive screening evaluation by a sleep specialist, a psychologist, and a physician to determine which ones were eligible. Fewer than half of the volunteers ultimately were found to be eligible.

Who Was Excluded: Patients whose insomnia was due to a medical condition or a medication, those with sleep apnea, those regularly taking sleep medications, those with a severe mental health disturbance, those living in a nursing home or other facility, and those with cognitive impairment.

How Many Patients: 78

Study Overview: See Figure 45.1 for a summary of the trial's design.

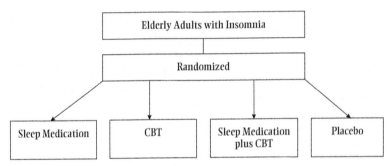

Figure 45.1 Summary of the Study Design.

Study Intervention: Patients assigned to receive CBT were offered weekly 90-minute group therapy sessions led by a clinical psychologist for 8 weeks. During these sessions, patients were taught to restrict time in bed in order to increase the proportion of time spent sleeping. In addition, patients were taught to use the bedroom only for sleep and to leave the bedroom whenever they could not fall asleep within 15–20 minutes. Finally, the CBT sessions addressed faulty beliefs about sleep (for example, that everyone must sleep 8 hours every night) and provided education about sleep hygiene and how sleep patterns change with normal aging.

Patients assigned to the medication group were prescribed temazepam to be taken 1 hour before bedtime. Patients met weekly with a psychiatrist to discuss medication management. The initial temazepam dose was 7.5 mg, and this could gradually be increased by the physician if necessary to a maximum of

30 mg. Patients were encouraged to use temazepam at least two to three nights per week and were given enough medication to use every night if they chose to.

Patients assigned to the combined CBT plus medication group received both of the above treatments.

Patients assigned to the placebo group received placebo pills according to the same schedule as patients in the temazepam group.

At the conclusion of the therapy, patients resumed regular treatment by their physician. However, follow-up monitoring continued for a total of 24 months.

Follow-Up: 24 months.

Endpoints: Sleep time as measured by sleep diaries kept by patients and by polysomnography, and scores on the Sleep Impairment Index, a survey that assesses the clinical severity of insomnia with respect to sleep disturbance, daytime functioning, distress caused by the sleep problem, and overall satisfaction with sleep.

RESULTS

- 63% of patients had mixed insomnia (i.e., both sleep-onset and sleep-maintenance insomnia), while 28% had only sleep-maintenance insomnia, and 6% had only sleep-onset insomnia.
- The average duration of insomnia symptoms among study patients was 17 years, and 77% of patients had previously used sleep medications.
- Treatment compliance in all groups was high: patients assigned to receive CBT attended 97% of the sessions, and patients assigned to receive medication took the medication approximately 75% of all nights.
- Sleep patterns as measured with sleep diaries improved with all three active treatments compared to placebo ($P < 0.05$; see Table 45.1).
- Sleep patterns as measured with polysomnography followed a similar pattern. However, only combined therapy resulted in statistically significant improvements compared to placebo (individually, CBT and medications resulted in nonsignificant improvements).
- The combined treatment appeared more effective than either CBT or medication individually; however, the difference did not reach statistical significance.

- CBT and combined treatment led to greater improvements on the patient-reported Sleep Impairment Index than did medication ($P = 0.01$) or placebo ($P = 0.002$).
- Improvements in sleep patterns were better sustained after 24 months with CBT than with pharmacotherapy.

Table 45.1 SUMMARY OF KEY FINDINGS

Total Sleep Time in Minutes[a]	CBT Group	Medication Group	Combined Therapy Group	Placebo Group
Pretreatment	322	340	290	331
Posttreatment	352	384	332	351
24-Month Follow-Up	387	352	331	331

[a] These data are from sleep diaries kept by patients. Polysomnography data followed a similar pattern.

Criticisms and Limitations: This study involved a carefully selected group of patients who were extremely compliant with the study protocol. These findings may not apply to patients outside of a research setting. For example, many real-world patients might not attend CBT sessions as reliably as these patients did.

In this study, CBT involved eight group sessions with a clinical psychologist. Such therapy may not be available in all settings, and it is also expensive.

For obvious reasons, neither the patients who received CBT nor their treating clinicians were blinded to the treatment assignment. It is possible that the lack of blinding could have biased the results. For example, patients in the CBT group may have been more likely to report improvements in their sleep patterns simply because they knew they were receiving a "real" treatment rather than placebo.

Because the sample size for this study was small (78 patients), the study was underpowered to detect small differences in the effectiveness of the three treatment options.

Other Relevant Studies and Information:

- Trials comparing CBT with medication for insomnia in both young adults and the elderly have generally come to similar conclusions as this trial.[2–4]
- In a trial comparing CBT with CBT combined with medication (zolpidem), the combined treatment led to a slightly better initial

response than CBT alone. However, patients in the combined group who were ultimately tapered off medication had the best response.[5]

- An analysis suggested higher rates of mortality among patients receiving common sleep medications. However, this was not a randomized trial and thus it does not prove that medications lead to increased mortality.[6]

- Most experts recommend CBT, either alone or (in severe cases) in combination with medication as first-line treatment for chronic insomnia; when medication is used, it should ideally only be given for several weeks.

Summary and Implications: All three treatments—CBT, medication, and combination therapy—improved symptoms of insomnia more than placebo. Combination therapy initially appeared to be most effective. However, both combination therapy and CBT alone led to greater improvements in patient-reported symptoms than medication alone. Importantly, CBT appeared to produce the best outcomes with long-term follow-up.

CLINICAL CASE: INSOMNIA IN THE ELDERLY

Case History:

A 76-year-old woman presents to your office 2 weeks after her husband unexpectedly passed away to ask if you can do anything to help with her insomnia. Upon further questioning, you discover that she has had trouble sleeping for several years, but the problem has become acutely worse since her husband died. She reports that she "hasn't slept a wink" in over a week, and she constantly feels tired and irritable during the day. In addition, the woman appears sad.

Based on the results of this trial, how should you treat her insomnia?

Suggested Answer:

This patient has chronic insomnia that has become acutely worse since her husband passed away. Given her acute psychological distress, it would be important to monitor her psychological state closely, particularly since elderly patients like her are prone to depression. You might suggest that she come for regular clinic visits or telephone consultations during this difficult time, or even refer her for formal counseling. In addition, you might encourage her to spend time with family and friends if possible.

For managing the insomnia, it would be preferable to avoid using a medi-cation and instead focus on behavioral modifications, including referral for CBT. Specifically, she might try using the bedroom only to sleep, leaving the bedroom when she has difficulty falling asleep, improving her sleep hygiene, and restricting her time in bed. Such treatment will ultimately have a more lasting impact on her sleep patterns than medication.

If this strategy is not successful, or if the patient strongly prefers to try a medication for this acute period, it would not be unreasonable to prescribe a low-dose sleep medication such as a benzodiazepine or zolpidem for a short period of time. However, if provided, these medications should be used extremely cautiously because elderly patients are prone to side effects such as oversedation.

References

1. Morin CM et al. Behavioral and pharmacological therapies for late-life insomnia: a randomized controlled trial. *JAMA*. 1999;281(11):991–999.
2. Jacobs GD et al. Cognitive behavior therapy and pharmacotherapy for insom-nia: a randomized controlled trial and direct comparison. *Arch Intern Med*. 2004;164(17):1888–1896.
3. Sivertsen B et al. Cognitive behavioral therapy vs. zopiclone for treatment of chronic primary insomnia in older adults. *JAMA*. 2006;295(24):2851–2858.
4. McClusky HY et al. Efficacy of behavioral vs. triazolam treatment in persistent sleep-onset insomnia. *Am J Psychiatry*. 1991;148(1):121–126.
5. Morin CM et al. Cognitive behavioral therapy, singly and combined with medication, for persistent insomnia: a randomized controlled trial. *JAMA*. 2009;301(19):2005.
6. Weich S et al. Effect of anxiolytic and hypnotic drug prescriptions on mortality hazards: retrospective cohort study. *BMJ*. 2014;348:g1996.

46

Treatment of Hypertension in the Elderly

The HYVET Trial

KRISTOPHER SWIGER

[Our result] provides unique evidence that hypertension treatment . . . in the very elderly . . . aimed to achieve a target blood pressure of 150/80 mmHg, is beneficial and is associated with reduced risks of death from stroke, death from any cause, and heart failure.

—BECKETT ET AL.[1]

Research Question: Is treatment of hypertension in patients who are over 80 years of age beneficial?[1]

Funding: The British Heart Foundation, a donation-based research and outreach organization, and the Servier Group, the maker of indapamide.

Year Study Began: 2000

Year Study Published: 2008

Study Location: 195 centers in Europe, China, Australasia, and Tunisia.

Who Was Studied: Patients ≥80 years of age with a history of hypertension who stopped all antihypertensive medications for a 2-month period and took one placebo pill daily. Patients were eligible for enrollment if, during this run-in period, they had a sustained systolic blood pressure of 160–199 mm Hg and a diastolic blood pressure <110 (at the start of the study, patients were also required to have a diastolic blood pressure ≥90; however, this requirement was relaxed partway through the study, allowing for inclusion of patients with isolated systolic hypertension).

Who Was Excluded: Patients with contraindications to the study medications or "heart failure requiring treatment with antihypertensive medications." Also excluded were patients with laboratory evidence of renal insufficiency, serum potassium outside of normal limits, or other conditions including gout, recent hemorrhagic stroke, or dementia. Patients with secondary hypertension were also excluded.

How Many Patients: 3,845

Study Overview: See Figure 46.1 for a summary of the design.

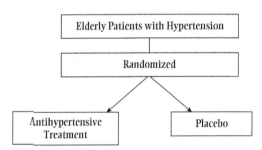

Figure 46.1 Summary of the Study Design.

Study Intervention: Patients in the active treatment arm were started on indapamide sustained release 1.5 mg (a thiazide-like diuretic) with the addition of perindopril 2 or 4 mg at the discretion of the treating physician to achieve a target blood pressure of <150/80. Patients in the placebo arm received matching placebo pills. Patients were withdrawn from the study if additional antihypertensive medications were used for more than 3 months or if blood pressure was >220/110 on two consecutive visits despite maximum treatment with the study drugs.

Follow-Up: Median of 1.8 years.

Endpoints: Primary outcome: Fatal or nonfatal stroke. Secondary outcomes: All-cause mortality, cardiovascular mortality, and fatal stroke.

RESULTS

- Baseline characteristics were similar between the two groups with an average age of 84 years; 61% of participants were female; and the average baseline blood pressure while sitting was 173/91.
- The study was terminated at the second interim analysis when a clear mortality benefit became apparent in the active treatment group.
- Blood pressure decreased in both groups but was more pronounced in the active treatment group, and a higher proportion of patients in the active treatment group met the blood pressure goal (<150/80; Table 46.1).
- Though there was a nonsignificant reduction in the incidence of strokes in the active treatment group compared to the placebo group at the time of publication, updated results published in 2012 found a significant reduction in strokes (21% reduction in fatal strokes) in the active treatment arm[2] (Table 46.1).
- All-cause mortality was 32% lower in the active treatment group relative to the placebo group (Table 46.1).
- There were no differences in potassium, uric acid, glucose, or creatinine levels between the groups.
- Serious adverse events were more common in the placebo group, and only five reported events (two in the active treatment group) were classified as related to the trial medications.

Table 46.1 SUMMARY OF KEY FINDINGS

Outcome	Active Treatment	Placebo	P Value
Mean Decrease in Seated Blood Pressure	−29.5/12.9 mm Hg	−14.5/6.8 mm Hg	not reported
Proportion of Patients Meeting Blood Pressure Goal (<150/80 mm Hg)	48.0%	19.9%	<0.001
Rate of Fatal and Nonfatal Strokes	11.7 per 1,000 person-years	17.3 per 1,000 person-years	0.04[a]
All-Cause Mortality	47.2 per 1,000 person-years	59.6 per 1,000 person-years	0.02
Rate of Fatal Stroke	6.5 per 1,000 person-years	10.7 per 1,000 person-years	0.046

[a] The figures reported for fatal and nonfatal strokes were those released in 2012 when additional data collected during the original study were released.

Criticisms and Limitations: The study population appeared to be healthier (lower rates of cardiovascular disease) than patients of similar age in the general population, and thus the results may not apply to the broader population. Additionally, adverse events were not clearly tracked or reported. For example, though patients were assessed for orthostatic hypotension with sitting and standing blood pressure measurements at each visit, the number of occurrences of orthostatic hypotension, a common side effect of antihypertensive medications in the elderly, was not reported.

Other Relevant Studies and Information:

- A meta-analysis of eight trials involving 15,693 patients demonstrated reduced cardiovascular morbidity and mortality in patients >60 years old with systolic blood pressure >160 mm Hg treated with antihypertensives compared to those left untreated. The greatest benefit was found among male patients and patients >70 years old.[3]
- The 2014 Evidence-Based Guideline for the Management of High Blood Pressure in Adults recommends the use of antihypertensive agents in the treatment of patients >60 years of age to target a blood pressure <150/90.[4]

Summary and Implications: The trial demonstrated an all-cause mortality benefit from the treatment of hypertension in patients >80 years old. Though a cautious approach is necessary, it appears that the benefits of hypertension treatment in the elderly outweigh the risks among carefully selected patients.

CLINICAL CASE: HYPERTENSION IN THE ELDERLY

Case History:

An 83-year-old man with a history of benign prostatic hypertrophy and hyperlipidemia presents for a routine follow-up. At previous examinations you noted his blood pressure was approximately 165/85 mm Hg. Currently, he is not taking any antihypertensive medications and his blood pressure is 170/76 while seated and 168/74 while standing.

As a next step, you recommend that he purchase a blood pressure cuff and take daily measurements at home for 2 weeks. When he returns, he provides a sheet of recorded values with an average systolic pressure of 170 mm Hg and an average diastolic pressure of 76 mm Hg. Based on the results of this trial, what is the best next step in the management of this patient's hypertension?

Suggested Answer:

This elderly patient has systolic hypertension and is similar to the patients enrolled in the study. As a first step, you might recommend lifestyle modification with weight loss, limited salt intake, and increased exercise. If the patient's blood pressure does not improve to an acceptable level, you should discuss the risks and benefits of antihypertensive medications with him. Specifically, you should inform him that, although antihypertensive medications have side effects such as orthostatic hypotension, fatigue, and electrolyte abnormalities, high-quality studies have demonstrated that treatment of hypertension in the elderly can reduce cardiovascular events and mortality rates. If the patient decides to proceed with medication therapy after understanding the risks and benefits, based on recommendations from guidelines, you might consider starting a thiazide diuretic, an angiotensin-converting enzyme inhibitor, or an angiotensin receptor blocker. When starting antihypertensives in elderly patients, you should monitor carefully for orthostatic hypotension and electrolyte abnormalities.

References

1. Beckett N et al. Treatment of hypertension in patients 80 years of age and older. *New Eng J Med*. 2008;358:1887–1898.
2. Beckett N et al. Immediate and late benefits of treating very elderly people with hypertension: results from the active treatment extension to hypertension in the very elderly randomised controlled trial. *BMJ*. 2012;doi:10:1136/bmj.d7541.
3. Staessen JA et al. Risks of untreated and treated isolated systolic hypertension in the elderly: meta-analysis of outcome trials. *Lancet*. 2000;355(9207):865.
4. James PA et al. 2014 Evidence-Based Guideline for the Management of High Blood Pressure in Adults: Report From the panel members appointed to the Eighth Joint National Committee (JNC 8). *JAMA*. 2013;(epub ahead of print):doi:10.1001/jama.2013.284427.

47

Use of Feeding Tubes in Patients with Dementia

STEVEN D. HOCHMAN

> The current study confirms the lack of treatment effect [from feeding-tube insertion] on survival [in patients with dementia].
>
> —TENO ET AL.[1]

Research Question: Does insertion of a percutaneous endoscopic gastrostomy (PEG) feeding tube in patients with dementia who need feeding assistance improve survival?[1]

Funding: The National Institute on Aging, part of the United States National Institute of Health.

Year Study Began: 1999

Year Study Published: 2012

Study Location: Nursing homes throughout the United States.

Who Was Studied: Medicare-enrolled patients in nursing homes with a diagnosis of dementia and first-time development of eating problems as determined by the Cognitive Performance Scale (CPS).

The CPS is a validated scale completed on all residents of Medicare- or Medicaid-certified nursing homes (a component of the Minimum Data Set). A change in score from 4 or 5 to 6 indicates that the patient has developed the need for assistance in eating. Patients were enrolled when they met eligibility criteria based on the CPS.

Approximately 5% of study patients received a PEG tube during the study period based on claims data and information from the Medicare Minimum Data Set. Since the decision about whether or not to insert a PEG tube was made at the discretion of the patient, his or her family, and the care team, this trial was not randomized.

Who Was Excluded: Patients in a coma, those with attempted feeding-tube insertion in the 6 months prior to enrollment, or those who died within 2 weeks of meeting eligibility criteria.

How Many Patients: 36,492, 5.4% of whom received PEG tubes

Study Overview: See Figure 47.1 for a summary of the study design.

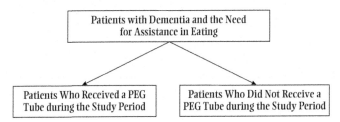

Figure 47.1 Summary of the Study Design.

Study Intervention: Patients in the PEG tube insertion group received a PEG tube during the study period while those in the control group did not. Patients in both groups were followed for 1 year or until death as ascertained from a Medicare database.

Follow-Up: 1 year or death, whichever came first.

Endpoints: Survival time, defined as the number of days from enrollment until the date of death. Survival time was adjusted for factors that may have confounded the results including sociodemographic characteristics, use of advanced care planning, concurrent medical diagnoses and clinical conditions (e.g., dehydration, infections), functional status, and two scores that predict mortality.

RESULTS

- The average age of study patients was 85 years and 78% were female.
- Feeding tubes were more likely to be placed in African American or Hispanic patients and those without documentation of advanced care planning.
- The average survival time among patients who received feeding tubes was 177 days and there was no significant difference in survival between patients with and without feeding-tube insertion (adjusted hazard ratio 1.03, 95% confidence interval 0.94–1.13).
- There was no difference in survival time between patients who underwent feeding-tube insertion within 4 months of enrollment and those with insertion >4 months after enrollment.

Criticisms and Limitations: The study was not a randomized trial, and despite rigorous attempts to adjust for potential confounding factors, the researchers may not have been able to control for everything. Specifically, patients who received feeding tubes may have been sicker than those who did not, despite the researchers' efforts to control for differences in morbidity between the groups. As a result, the benefits of PEG tube insertion may have been obscured.

Other Relevant Studies and Information:

- A systematic review of seven observational studies failed to demonstrate survival benefit from PEG feeding-tube insertion among patients with advanced dementia.[2]
- An observational study of 178 patients with advanced dementia found no difference in the level of discomfort between patients in whom artificial nutrition and hydration were initiated and those in whom this care was withheld.[3]
- In an analysis of hospitalized patients with advanced dementia and need for assistance in eating, PEG tube insertion did not reduce the risk of pressure ulcers or help existing pressure ulcers to heal.[4]
- There have not been any randomized trials evaluating the impact of PEG tube insertion among patients with dementia.
- The American Geriatrics Society position statement on the use of feeding tubes in older adults with advanced dementia recommends against the use of feeding tubes in favor of careful hand feeding.[5]

Summary and Implications: This study found that PEG tube insertion in patients with dementia and eating difficulties did not improve survival. In addition, the timing of feeding-tube insertion, early or late following the development of eating difficulties, did not affect survival. Because this study was not randomized, it is possible that unmeasured confounding factors obscured the benefits of feeding-tube placement. Still, based on this study and several others, the American Geriatrics Society recommends against the use of feeding tubes in older adults with advanced dementia.

CLINICAL CASE: FEEDING TUBES IN PATIENTS WITH DEMENTIA

Case History:

An 85-year-old man with a history of Alzheimer's disease is admitted to a nursing home with increasing difficulty in performing activities of daily living and worsening of short-term memory. At the time of admission, the patient is still able to feed himself without difficulty. Three months following admission, the patient has lost 8 pounds and has had increasing difficulty feeding himself, though he is still able to accomplish the task with intermittent help. Based on the results of this trial, how should this patient and his family be counseled at this time?

Suggested Answer:

Like many patients with dementia, this patient is experiencing increasing difficulties with eating and has resultant weight loss. Because he is still able to feed himself, he has not yet progressed to the most advanced stage of dementia based on the Cognitive Performance Assessment (and thus he would not have met the entry criteria for this study). However, he may progress to this stage soon. As you discuss goals of care with the patient and his family, you should inform them that existing data, though imperfect, do not suggest that feeding-tube insertion prolongs survival. Furthermore, other studies suggest that feeding-tube insertion does not improve comfort or other health outcomes. Because of these data, guidelines from the American Geriatrics Society recommend against PEG tube insertion in patients like this. This information should enable the patient and his family to make an informed decision about whether or not he should receive a PEG tube if his feeding difficulties progress.

References

1. Teno JM et al. Does feeding tube insertion and its timing improve survival? *J Am Geriatr Soc.* 2012;60:1918.
2. Sampson EL, Candy B, Jones L. Enteral tube feeding for older people with advanced dementia. *Cochrane Database Syst Rev.* 2009:CD007209.
3. Pasman HR et al. Discomfort in nursing home patients with severe dementia in whom artificial nutrition and hydration is forgone. *Arch Intern Med.* 2005;165:1729.
4. Teno JM et al. Feeding tubes and the prevention or healing of pressure ulcers. *Arch Intern Med.* 2012;172:697.
5. American Geriatrics Society Executive Committee. Feeding tubes in advanced dementia position statement. May 2013. http://www.americangeriatrics.org/files/documents/feeding.tubes.advanced.dementia.pdf

48

Early Palliative Care in Non-Small-Cell Lung Cancer

MICHAEL E. HOCHMAN

Early integration of palliative care with standard oncologic care in patients with metastatic non-small-cell lung cancer resulted in survival that was prolonged by approximately 2 months and clinically meaningful improvements in quality of life and mood.

—TEMEL ET AL.[1]

Research Question: Can early palliative care improve the quality of life of patients with metastatic non-small-cell lung cancer (NSCLC)? Also, what is the impact of early palliative care on survival?[1]

Funding: An American Society of Clinical Oncology Career Development Award, as well as gifts from two cancer foundations.

Year Study Began: 2006

Year Study Published: 2010

Study Location: One university-affiliated hospital in the United States.

Who Was Studied: Patients in the ambulatory care setting with metastatic NSCLC diagnosed within the previous 8 weeks. In addition, patients were required to have an Eastern Cooperative Oncology Group performance status of 0, 1, or 2 (0 = asymptomatic; 1 = symptomatic but fully ambulatory; and 2 = symptomatic and in bed <50% of the day).

Who Was Excluded: Patients who were already receiving palliative care services.

How Many Patients: 151

Study Overview: See Figure 48.1 for a summary of the trial's design.

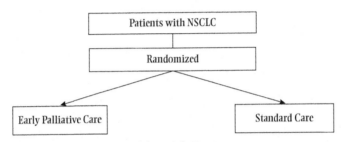

Figure 48.1 Summary of the Study Design.

Study Intervention: Patients in the early palliative care group met with a palliative care physician or nurse within 3 weeks of enrollment and at least monthly thereafter. Additional palliative care visits could be scheduled as needed. The palliative care visits focused on assessing emotional and physical symptoms, establishing goals of care, and coordinating care.

Patients in the standard-care group received palliative care visits only when meetings were requested by the patient, the family, or the oncologist.

Patients in both groups received standard cancer therapy throughout the study.

Follow-Up: 12 weeks for the primary analysis; over a year for the survival analysis.

Endpoints: Primary outcome: Change from baseline to 12 weeks in quality-of-life scores, which were measured using components of the Functional Assessment of Cancer Therapy-Lung (FACT-L) scale. The components of the scale that were used included physical and functional well-being, as well as "seven symptoms specific to lung cancer." Secondary outcomes: Depression, as assessed by the Hospital Anxiety and Depression scale and the Patient Health Questionnaire 9; healthcare utilization; documentation of resuscitation preferences; and survival.

RESULTS

- Patients in the early palliative care group received an average of four palliative care visits.
- 14% of patients in the standard-care group received a palliative care consultation during the first 12 weeks of the study.
- Early palliative care had favorable effects on quality of life and depression and prolonged survival (see Table 48.1).

Table 48.1 SUMMARY OF KEY FINDINGS

Outcome	Early Palliative Care Group	Standard-Care Group	P Value
Change in Quality-of-Life Scores[a]	+2.3	−2.3	0.04
Symptoms of Depression[b]	16%	38%	0.01
Aggressive End-of-Life Care[c]	33%	54%	0.05
Documentation of Resuscitation Preferences	53%	28%	0.05
Median Survival	11.6 months	8.9 months	0.02

[a] Scores on the scale range from 0 to 84 with higher scores indicating a better quality of life. At baseline, the mean score in the early palliative care group was 56.2 versus 55.3 in the standard-care group.
[b] As assessed using the Hospital Anxiety and Depression Scale. A similar pattern was seen when depression was assessed using the Patient Health Questionnaire 9.
[c] The authors classified patients as having received aggressive end-of-life care if they received chemotherapy within 14 days of death, did not receive hospice care, or were admitted to hospice within 3 days of death.

Criticisms and Limitations: It is not clear whether the benefits of early palliative care resulted from particular components of the intervention or whether the benefits resulted from additional time and attention from the palliative care team.

Other Relevant Studies and Information:

- A follow-up qualitative analysis of this study demonstrated that the palliative care visits provided to the intervention group emphasized "managing symptoms, strengthening coping, and cultivating illness understanding and prognostic awareness."[2]
- The ENABLE II trial showed that a palliative care intervention in patients with advanced cancer led to improvements in quality of life and mood, but not to improvements in symptom intensity or a

reduction in hospital or emergency room visits.[3] A post hoc analysis did not show a significant effect of the intervention on survival (median survival was 14 months in the palliative care group versus 8.5 months for the standard-care group, $P = 0.14$).[3] The ENABLE II intervention was largely telephone-based.

- Because of mounting data demonstrating the benefits of early palliative care, a recent provisional clinical opinion from the American Society of Clinical Oncology recommends early palliative care for most patients with metastatic cancer and/or high symptom burden.[4]

Summary and Implications: Palliative care consultation soon after the diagnosis of NSCLC has beneficial effects on quality of life and symptoms of depression, and it also appears to prolong survival. Early palliative care is an appropriate component of standard therapy for NSCLC and perhaps other advanced cancers.

CLINICAL CASE: EARLY PALLIATIVE CARE CONSULTATION

Case History:
A 74-year-old woman is diagnosed with metastatic ovarian cancer. She is seen in your oncology clinic for an initial consultation 2 weeks later. In addition to discussing her therapeutic options, should you refer this patient for a palliative care consultation?

Suggested Answer:
Although this trial only involved patients with NSCLC, it demonstrated the value of palliative care services in improving quality of life and symptoms of depression in patients with advanced cancer. In addition, early palliative care consultation was associated with prolonged survival.

Metastatic ovarian cancer, like metastatic NSCLC, has a poor prognosis: patients with stage III or IV ovarian cancer have a 5-year survival rate of less than 50%. While no well-designed trials have evaluated the impact of early palliative care among patients with metastatic ovarian cancer, based on the results of this trial it is likely that early palliative care is beneficial. Thus, it would be quite appropriate to refer this patient to a palliative care specialist who could help manage your patient's emotional and physical symptoms and could help to establish realistic goals of care. (Note that palliative care is not synonymous with hospice. Hospice is designed for patients at the end of life whose primary goal is comfort rather than extending life. Palliative care is designed to improve quality of life among patients with serious illnesses who frequently are receiving therapy aimed at extending—or curing—a disease.)

References

1. Temel JS et al. Early palliative care for patients with metastatic non-small-cell lung cancer. *N Engl J Med*. 2010;363(8):733–742.
2. Yoong J et al. Early palliative care in advanced lung cancer: a qualitative study. *JAMA Intern Med*. 2013;173(4):283–290.
3. Bakitas M et al. Effects of a palliative care intervention on clinical outcomes in patients with advanced cancer: the Project ENABLE II randomized controlled trial. *JAMA*. 2009;302(7):741–749.
4. Smith TJ et al. American Society of Clinical Oncology provisional clinical opinion: the integration of palliative care into standard oncology care. *J Clin Oncol*. 2012;30(8):880.

SECTION 11

Mental Health

49

Initial Treatment of Depression

MICHAEL E. HOCHMAN

> [Patients] have an equal probability of recovering from [depression] whether treated pharmacologically or psychotherapeutically, even though the clinical progress will likely be slower with [psychotherapy].
> —SCHULBERG ET AL.[1]

Research Question: Is pharmacotherapy or psychotherapy more effective for the treatment of depression? Also, are these treatments superior to usual depression care from primary care doctors?[1]

Funding: The National Institute of Mental Health.

Year Study Began: 1991

Year Study Published: 1996

Study Location: Four outpatient clinics affiliated with the University of Pittsburgh.

Who Was Studied: Patients 18–64 who fulfilled DSM-III-R criteria[2] for current major depression and who had a minimum score of 13 on the 17-item Hamilton Rating Scale-Depression (HRS-D).[3] These determinations were made by a psychiatrist.

The HRS-D scale is described below. The DSM-III-R criteria for depression, which are similar to the DSM-IV criteria, include the presence of dysphoria along with most of the following other symptoms:

- loss of interest
- appetite disturbance
- sleep disturbance
- psychomotor change
- loss of energy
- feelings of guilt
- slowed thinking or concentration disturbance
- thoughts of death or suicide

Who Was Excluded: Patients with another medical or psychiatric condition preventing random assignment to one of the treatment groups. In addition, patients receiving current treatment for a mood disorder were ineligible.

How Many Patients: 276

Study Overview: See Figure 49.1 for a summary of the trial's design.

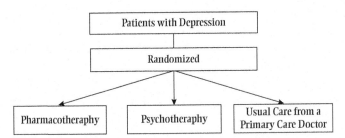

Figure 49.1 Summary of the Study Design.

Study Intervention: Patients assigned to receive pharmacotherapy were treated with nortriptyline by family practitioners or general internists trained in pharmacotherapy. Each patient was treated within his or her regular medical clinic; however, the prescribing doctor was not the patient's usual doctor. Patients were initially started on a nortriptyline dose of 25 mg and were seen weekly or every 2 weeks for medication titration. Once patients showed clinical improvement and had therapeutic nortriptyline serum levels (190– 570 nmol/L), they were transitioned to monthly visits for an additional 6 months.

Patients assigned to psychotherapy were treated with interpersonal psycho-therapy by psychiatrists and psychologists. Patients received 16 weekly sessions at their regular medical clinic followed by four monthly maintenance sessions.

Patients assigned to usual care were treated by their primary care physicians according to each physician's regular practices.

Follow-Up: 8 months.

Endpoints: Mean scores on the HRS-D. In addition, the authors determined the proportion of patients in each group who had "recovered" from depression as indicated by an HRS-D score ≤7.

The HRS-D is a commonly used depression scoring system based on the severity of depression symptoms. It is administered by clinicians. A score ≥20 is commonly considered to indicate depression of moderate severity. Study patients were required to have a minimum HSR-D score of 13, and the mean baseline score of study patients was 23. Below is a sample item on the 17-item survey:

- Depressed Mood:
  0-absent
  1-these feeling states indicated only on questioning
  2-these feelings states spontaneously reported verbally
  3-communicates feeling states nonverbally, that is, through facial
     expressions, posture, voice, and tendency to weep
  4-patient reports virtually only these feeling states in his/her
     spontaneous verbal and nonverbal communication

RESULTS

- The mean age of study patients was 38, and more than 80% were female.
- The mean baseline HRS-D score for study patients was 23.
- 33% of patients assigned to pharmacotherapy completed all 8 months of therapy versus 42% of patients assigned to psychotherapy.
- In the usual care group, 63% of patients received some form of mental health treatment and 45% received an antidepressant within 2 months of the trial's onset.
- Both nortriptyline and psychotherapy were more effective than usual care. However, there were no significant differences in depression symptoms between patients assigned to nortriptyline versus psychotherapy (see Table 49.1).

- Improvement was more rapid among patients receiving nortriptyline versus psychotherapy (not shown in Table 49.1).

Table 49.1 SUMMARY OF KEY FINDINGS

Outcome	Nortriptyline Group	Psychotherapy Group	Usual Care Group	Significance Testing[a]
Mean HRS-D Score at Trial Completion	9.0	9.3	13.1	Nortriptyline and psychotherapy were superior to usual care; there was no difference between nortriptyline and psychotherapy.
Depression Recovery Rate (HRS-D ≤7)	48%	46%	18%	Nortriptyline and psychotherapy were superior to usual care; there was no difference between nortriptyline and psychotherapy.

[a] Actual *P* values not reported.

Criticisms and Limitations: Primary care doctors treating patients assigned to the usual care group were not always informed immediately that their patients had been diagnosed with depression. This may have caused a delay in treatment initiation, potentially leading to poorer outcomes among patients in the usual care group.

Depression therapies have evolved since this trial was conducted. For example, selective serotonin reuptake inhibitors (SSRIs)—not nortriptyline—are now first-line pharmacotherapy for depression due to their more favorable side-effect profile.[4] More recent trials comparing SSRIs with psychotherapy have come to similar conclusions as this one, however.[5,6]

Finally, just 33% of patients assigned to pharmacotherapy and 42% of patients assigned to psychotherapy completed all 8 months of therapy. This demonstrates the challenges of treating patients with depression with either of these modalities.

Other Relevant Studies and Information:

- Other trials comparing antidepressant medications with psychotherapy have come to similar conclusions as this one.[5-8]
- Some studies have suggested that a combination of pharmacotherapy and psychotherapy may be slightly more beneficial than either treatment alone, particularly for patients with severe chronic depression.[9]
- Guidelines from the Agency for Health Care Policy and Research conclude that either medication or psychotherapy is an appropriate initial therapy for mild or moderate depression. However, severely depressed patients should receive medications.[10]

Summary and Implications: In primary care patients with depression, initial treatment with psychotherapy or pharmacotherapy (nortriptyline) was equally efficacious; however, clinical improvement was slightly faster with pharmacotherapy. The psychotherapy and pharmacotherapy protocols used in this trial were both superior to usual care from primary care doctors, highlighting the need for standardized depression treatment.

CLINICAL CASE: INITIAL TREATMENT OF DEPRESSION

Case History:

A 52-year-old woman visits your primary care office because she has been feeling "down" for the past 2 months. She says that life's stresses have been wearing on her. She has had several previous depressive episodes but has never sought medical attention before. She reports that she has not been sleeping well, her energy level has been low, and she frequently feels guilty and inadequate. She denies problems with her appetite, psychomotor changes, difficulty concentrating, suicidal ideations, or frequent thoughts of death.

Based on the results of this trial, what treatment options would you consider for this patient?

Suggested Answer:

This trial demonstrated that psychotherapy and pharmacotherapy were equally efficacious for the initial management of depression; however, clinical improvement was slightly faster with pharmacotherapy.

The patient in this vignette has symptoms consistent with mild depression. She could be treated with either psychotherapy—assuming high-quality psychotherapy services are available—or pharmacotherapy (likely an SSRI because of the favorable side-effects profile). After explaining the options to the patient, you should ask which approach she prefers.

References

1. Schulberg HC et al. Treating major depression in primary care practice. *Arch Gen Psychiatry.* 1996;53:913–919.
2. American Psychiatric Association. *Diagnostic and statistical manual of mental disorders,* Third Edition, Revised. Washington, DC: Author, 1987.
3. Hamilton M. A rating scale for depression. *J Neurol Neurosurg Psychiatry.* 1960;23:56–62.
4. Mulrow CD et al. Efficacy of newer medications for treating depression in primary care patients. *Am J Med.* 2000;108(1):54.
5. Chilvers C et al. Antidepressant drugs and generic counseling for treatment of major depression in primary care: randomized trial with patient preference arms. *BMJ.* 2001;322:1–5.
6. DeRubeis RJ et al. Cognitive therapy vs. medications in the treatment of moderate to severe depression. *Arch Gen Psychiatry.* 2005;62:409–416.
7. Schulberg HC et al. The effectiveness of psychotherapy in treating depressive disorders in primary care practice: clinical and cost perspectives. *Gen Hosp Psychiatry.* 2002;24(4):203.
8. Cuijpers P et al. The efficacy of psychotherapy in treating depressive and anxiety disorders: a meta-analysis of direct comparisons. *World Psychiatry.* 2013 June;12(2):137–148.
9. Pampallona S et al. Combined pharmacotherapy and psychological treatment for depression: a systematic review. *Arch Gen Psychiatry.* 2004;61(7):714.
10. Depression Guideline Panel. *Depression in primary care: treatment of major depression: clinical practice guideline.* US Dept. of Health and Human Services, Public Health Service, Agency for Health Care Policy and Research. AHCPR publication 93-0551, Rockville, MD 1993.

50

Symptom-Triggered versus Fixed-Dose Therapy for Alcohol Withdrawal

KRISTOPHER SWIGER

[For patients experiencing alcohol withdrawal,] symptom-triggered therapy [with benzodiazepines] ... decreases both treatment duration and the amount of benzodiazepine used, and is as efficacious as standard fixed-schedule therapy for alcohol withdrawal.

—SAITZ ET AL.[1]

Research Question: In patients with alcohol withdrawal, should benzodiazepines be prescribed based on signs and symptoms or on a set, fixed-dose schedule?[1]

Funding: Roche Laboratories supplied the chlordiazepoxide used in the study.

Year Study Began: 1992

Year Study Published: 1994

Study Location: One alcohol detoxification unit in the United States.

Who Was Studied: Adults with an alcohol use disorder admitted to the Veterans Affairs Medical Center Alcohol Detoxification Unit for treatment of alcohol withdrawal.

Who Was Excluded: Patients with "concurrent acute medical or psychiatric illness requiring hospitalization," those with a history of seizures, and those unable to take oral medications. Also excluded were those with "current use of or withdrawal from opiates, benzodiazepines, barbiturates, clonidine, or beta blockers."

How Many Patients: 101

Study Overview: See Figure 50.1 for a summary of the study's design.

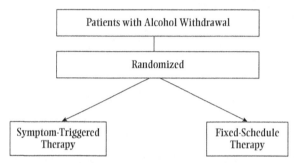

Figure 50.1 Summary of the Study Design.

Study Intervention: Patients in both groups were assessed for the severity of alcohol withdrawal on admission and every 8 hours thereafter. Patients were also assessed 1 hour after administration of benzodiazepines. Assessment was completed using the Clinical Institute Withdrawal Assessment for Alcohol, revised (CIWA-Ar) scale, with scores ranging from 0 to 67 (Box 50.1).

Box 50.1 CLINICAL INSTITUTE WITHDRAWAL ASSESSMENT FOR ALCOHOL

Each of the following is graded on a scale of 0–7 (0 is none and 7 is most severe):

- Nausea and vomiting
- Autonomic hyperactivity (pulse rate or sweating)
- Anxiety
- Agitation
- Tremor
- Headache

- Auditory disturbances
- Visual disturbances
- Tactile disturbances
- Sensorium (assessed on a scale of 0–4 where 0 is oriented and 4 is completely disoriented)

The individual scores are summed to produce a summary score.

Patients in the "fixed-schedule group received chlordiazepoxide every 6 hours for 12 doses" regardless of their CIWA-Ar score starting at admission (four doses of 50 mg each followed by eight doses of 25 mg each). Scheduled doses were not given if the patient was somnolent or refused medication. In addition, patients whose CIWA-Ar score was ≥8 were given additional doses of chlordiazepoxide ranging from 25 to 100 mg (the dose was at the treating nurse's discretion). This protocol was continued until the fixed-dosing schedule was complete and the patient's CIWA-Ar score was below 8 without medication.

Patients in the symptom-triggered group were given chlordiazepoxide only if their CIWA-Ar score was ≥8. Again, the dose ranged from 25 to 100 mg at the treating nurse's discretion. The protocol was continued until the patient's CIWA-Ar score was below 8 without medication.

Follow-Up: 30 days following hospital discharge.

Endpoints: Primary outcomes: Duration of time from admission to last dose of benzodiazepines required as well as the total dose of benzodiazepines administered. Secondary outcomes: Number of times benzodiazepines were administered in response to symptoms and median dose for these administrations; severity of alcohol withdrawal; proportion of patients leaving the hospital against medical advice; composite of development of hallucinations, seizures, or delirium tremens; and rates of rehabilitation, readmission, and compliance with follow-up.

RESULTS

- Medication treatment duration and the dose of benzodiazepine were lower in the symptom-triggered group compared with the fixed-schedule group (Table 50.1).

- The median number of symptom-triggered doses and the quantity of benzodiazepine delivered in these doses were similar between the two groups (Table 50.1).
- There were no between-group differences in patients leaving the hospital against medical advice or in the incidence of seizures, hallucinations, or delirium tremens.
- Patients in both groups were equally likely to be readmitted for alcohol withdrawal within 30 days and equally likely to enter rehabilitation or maintain compliance with outpatient treatment following discharge.

Table 50.1 SUMMARY OF KEY FINDINGS

Outcome	Symptom-Triggered Group	Fixed-Schedule Group	P Value
Duration of Treatment (Median)	9 hours	68 hours	<0.001
Total Dose of Benzodiazepine (Median)	100 mg	425 mg	<0.001
Number of Symptom-Triggered Doses (Median)	2	2	nonsignificant[a]
Amount of Symptom-Triggered Doses (Median)	100 mg	163 mg	nonsignificant[a]
Highest CIWA-Ar Score (Mean)	11	11	0.73

[a] Actual *P* value not reported, though $P > 0.05$ in both cases.

Criticisms and Limitations: The study excluded patients with current or past seizures, concurrent medical or psychiatric illnesses, and those concurrently using or withdrawing from other drugs and medications, which may limit the generalizability of the results. Patients with a history of or current seizures in particular may benefit from at least a single scheduled administration of benzodiazepines to prevent recurrent seizures.[2]

Furthermore, the study was conducted in an alcohol detoxification unit with specially trained nurses, raising questions about whether this approach would apply in other settings. Finally, the study had limited power to detect differences in several of the secondary outcomes such as leaving the hospital against medical advice or compliance with follow-up.

Other Relevant Studies and Information:

- Several other studies conducted in the emergency department,[3] on medical wards,[4] and in alcohol treatment units[5] are consistent with the findings of this trial.
- The American Society of Addiction Medicine guidelines recommend using benzodiazepines in alcohol withdrawal on a symptom-triggered basis.[6]

Summary and Implications: For patients with alcohol withdrawal, symptom-triggered benzodiazepine therapy was as effective as fixed-schedule therapy and led to a shorter duration of therapy and a lower total dose of benzodiazepines. These results may only apply to patients who are able to report symptoms and are cared for on a unit equipped to serially assess signs and symptoms of withdrawal. Even so, symptom-triggered benzodiazepine therapy is now the preferred strategy for patients presenting with alcohol withdrawal.

CLINICAL CASE: ALCOHOL WITHDRAWAL

Case History:

A 54-year-old man with a history of chronic obstructive pulmonary disease (COPD), severe alcohol use disorder, and a history of alcohol withdrawal presents with a COPD exacerbation. On his initial exam he is breathing comfortably on 2 liters nasal cannula with minimal wheezing. He reports his last drink as 24 hours prior to admission and he is concerned that he is starting to feel "shaky" and "anxious." You suspect he is experiencing symptoms of alcohol withdrawal.

Based on the results of the trial, what is the most appropriate strategy to treat his withdrawal?

Suggested Answer:

This study found that symptom-triggered benzodiazepine therapy was as effective as fixed-schedule therapy and led to a shorter duration of therapy and a lower total dose of benzodiazepines. The patient in this vignette is typical of those included in this study. Thus, it would be preferable to treat him with symptom-triggered therapy rather than fixed-dose therapy, ideally in a setting where staff are well trained in assessing alcohol withdrawal.

References

1. Saitz R et al. Individualized treatment for alcohol withdrawal: a randomized double-blind controlled trial. *JAMA.* 1994;272:519.
2. D'Onofrio G et al. Lorazepam for the prevention of recurrent seizures related to alcohol. *N Engl J Med.* 1999;340(12):915–919.
3. Cassidy EM et al. Symptom-triggered benzodiazepine therapy for alcohol withdrawal syndrome in the emergency department: a comparison with the standard fixed dose benzodiazepine regimen. *Emerg Med J.* 2012;29:802.
4. Jaeger TM, Lohr RH, Pankratz VS. Symptom-triggered therapy for alcohol withdrawal syndrome in medical inpatients. *Mayo Clin Proc.* 2001;76:695.
5. Daeppen JB et al. Symptom-triggered vs fixed-schedule doses of benzodiazepine for alcohol withdrawal: a randomized treatment trial. *Arch Intern Med.* 2002;162:1117.
6. Mayo-Smith MF. Pharmacologic management of alcohol withdrawal. A meta-analysis and evidence-based practice guideline. American Society of Addiction Medicine Working Group on Pharmacologic Management of Alcohol Withdrawal. *JAMA.* 1997;278(2):144–151.

Index

Page numbers followed by t indicate a table.

CPSIA information can be obtained
at www.ICGtesting.com
Printed in the USA
BVOW08s0046101217

502178BV00002B/7/P